Market-Driven Nursing

Developing and Marketing Patient Care Services

AONE Leadership Series

American Organization of Nurse Executives

Health Forum, Inc.
An American Hospital Association Company
CHICAGO

Printed in the United States of America—1/99

Cover design by Lori Buley

Library of Congress Cataloging-in-Publication Data

Market-driven nursing : developing and marketing patient care services
   / by American Organization of Nurse Executives.
      p.   cm. — (AONE leadership series)
   Includes index.
   ISBN 1-55648-247-7
   1. Nursing services—Marketing.   I. American Organization of
Nurse Executives.   II. Series.
RT86.7.M38   1999
362.1'73'0688—dc21   98-45912
                                                                          CIP

Item Number: 154155

Contents

iii

About the Editor

Judith A. Ryan, PhD, FAAN, is president and chief executive officer of the Evangelical Lutheran Good Samaritan Society. Formerly, she was associate director of the University of Iowa Hospitals and Clinics, senior vice president and chief quality officer of Lutheran General Health System, and executive director of the American Nurses Association. She has provided nurse-executive leadership on a number of strategic initiatives that have responded to unmet market demand for nursing services, including the National Center for Nursing Research, community nursing organizations, parish nursing, Congregational Health Services, the American Academy of Nursing's Expert Panel on Quality of Care, and the University of Iowa Nursing Enterprise. Dr. Ryan holds a BSN from St. Olaf College and a PhD in hospital and health care administration from the University of Minnesota. She is a fellow of the American Academy of Nursing.

About the Authors

Martha Boysen, MA, is a program associate in the Department of Nursing and Patient Care Services at the University of Iowa Hospitals and Clinics in Iowa City, Iowa. She received her master's degree in English from Iowa State University.

Karen Brugler, MM, LCSW, is a consultant in the health care consulting practice of Ernst & Young LLP. Former director of quality management at Lutheran General Hospital in Park Ridge, Illinois, she designed and implemented several innovative programs and services there, including the Laureate Day School for Emotionally Disturbed Children, the SPIRIT Employee Recognition Program, the Outpatient Anticoagulation Clinic, the Health and Happiness Lecture Series, and the Diagnostic Breast Center. Ms. Brugler holds a master's degree in social work from Jane Adams College of Social Work and a master of management degree from J. L. Kellogg Graduate School of Management.

Lois Evans, DNSc, RN, FAAN, is professor and Viola MacInnes/Independence Chair in Nursing, University of Pennsylvania School of Nursing, where she directs the school's academic nursing practices. Formerly, she directed one of the 11 Robert Wood Johnson Foundation Teaching Nursing Home projects. She holds an undergraduate degree in nursing from West Virginia University, masters and doctoral degrees in psychiatric–mental health nursing from The Catholic University of America, Washington, DC, and a certificate in primary care of older adults from the University of Rochester. Dr. Evans is a fellow of the American Academy of Nursing and the Gerontological Society of America.

Beverly Folkedahl, RN, CWOCN, developed the University of Iowa Department of Nursing's specialty practice in wound, ostomy, and continence nursing (WOCN) services. She is an advanced practice nurse certified in wound ostomy continence nursing and serves as clinical preceptor for WOC nursing education programs throughout the country. She has chaired the WOCN Ostomy DMERC Reimbursement Committee since 1994.

Kristine M. Gebbie, DrPH, RN, is the Elizabeth Standish Gill Associate Professor of Nursing and director, Center for Health Policy and Health Services Research at Columbia University School of Nursing. Her teaching and research focus is health policy and services, particularly population-based public health services. She also serves as a senior consultant on public health initiatives to the Office of Public Health and Science, U.S. Department of Health and Human Services. Dr. Gebbie was appointed by President Clinton to serve as the first national AIDS policy coordinator and was also a member of the Presidential Commission on AIDS. Dr. Gebbie has served as secretary of the Department of Health for the state of Washington and public health administrator for the state of Oregon. She has been active in many professional organizations and has served as a member of the executive board of the American Public Health Association. Her recent publications include a chapter on community-based care in *Information Networks for Community Health*, edited by Brennan, Schneider, and Tornquist. Dr. Gebbie has a bachelor of science degree in nursing from St. Olaf College, a masters of nursing from the University of California at Los Angeles, and a doctorate of public health in health policy from the University of Michigan School of Public Health.

Jody Kurtt, RN, MA, is associate director for nursing, Children's and Women's Services, at the University of Iowa Hospitals and Clinics. She has more than 20 years of nursing experience in clinical and administrative positions, focusing on children's and women's health care. Ms. Kurtt received a bachelor of science in nursing from Coe College, her master of arts in nursing from the University of Iowa, and is certified both as a pediatric nurse practitioner and in advanced nursing administration.

Gerri S. Lamb, PhD, RN, FAAN, is senior corporate director for community services at Carondelet Health Network in Tucson. She has been associated with Carondelet's innovative community-based nursing programs for a decade and has directed Carondelet's Community Nursing Organization (CNO) since its inception in 1994. She has published extensively on community case management and nursing care delivery systems. She has been on numerous professional committees and task force groups on payment for nursing services and managed care. She recently co-authored a work, *Case Management: A Guide to Strategic Evaluation*, that addresses developing practical systems for performance management. She is a fellow in the American Academy of Nursing. Dr. Lamb received her master's degree in the adult nurse practitioner program at the University of Rochester and her doctorate in clinical nursing research from the University of Arizona.

Norma M. Lang, PhD, RN, FAAN, FRCN, is the Margaret Bond Simon Dean and Professor at the University of Pennsylvania School of

Nursing. The seminal model for measuring and evaluating the quality of nursing care that bears her name has been adopted in the United States, Canada, Australia, and the United Kingdom. She chaired the ANA Congress on Nursing Practice, which issued "Nursing: A Social Policy Statement," and the Steering Committee on Data Bases for Clinical Practice. She serves as a consultant to the International Council of Nurses for the development of an International Classification of Nursing Practice. Dr. Lang is a fellow of the Institute of Medicine, the American Academy of Nursing, and the College of Physicians of Philadelphia and an honorary fellow of the Royal College of Nursing in London. She received her BSN from Alverno College, Milwaukee, and her MSN and PhD from Marquette University.

Mary Anne McCrea, MS, RN, CNA, ACHE, is the senior corporate director, patient care services, of Carondelet Health Network, Tucson. Since 1971 she has worked in an acute-care setting with a clinical specialty of critical care, and she has worked around Phoenix and Tucson (an area known for leadership in moving into managed care markets) throughout her 26-year career. She is affiliated with Sigma Theta Tau International Beta Upsilon Chapter, Arizona State Nurses Association, Arizona Organization of Nurse Executives. She also has an associate status in the American College of Healthcare Executives, is a member of the American Nurses Association Managed Care Working Group, and has been a member of the Carondelet Community Trust Council since 1997. Ms. McCrea has authored and co-authored several articles for health care publications. Most recently, her contributions have appeared in the journal *Seminars for Nurse Managers* and in *Nurses and Work Satisfaction: An Index for Measurement,* published by Health Administration Press.

Mae Taylor Moss, MS, MSN, RN, FAAN, founder of Moss Management, is a consultant and author. She has assisted medical and surgical services as well as administrative departments across the United States and Central America, Russia, Australia, and Tasmania to restructure health care processes. Former vice president for perioperative services at St. Luke's Hospital in Houston, she developed a myriad of cutting edge programs such as the Registered Nurse First Assistant and the Continuous Quality Improvement and Safety Programs, which lead the nation in positive patient outcomes. Ms. Moss is the author of the book *Reengineering of Operative and Invasive Services,* and is a frequent lecturer and contributor to professional journals on topics related to outcomes management, collaborative care, restructuring, and managed care issues. She is a fellow in the American Academy of Nursing.

Laurence J. O'Connell, PhD, STD, president and CEO of the Park Ridge Center for Health, Faith and Ethics, affiliate of Advocate Health

Care System, was awarded the prestigious Golden Eurydice Award in the Danish Parliament in 1996 for "his persistent work in organizing structures for bioethical debate and exceptional contributions to the understanding of sound ethical reasoning." Prior to assuming the presidency of Park Ridge Center, Dr. O'Connell was director of theology, mission, and ethics at the Catholic Health Association of the United States. He was an international adviser to the Commission of the European Community and the Council of Europe and served on the ethics working group of President Clinton's Task Force on National Health Care Reform. He holds a doctorate in religious studies and an STD in theology from the University of Louvain, Belgium.

Tim Porter-O'Grady, EdD, PhD, FAAN, is founder and senior partner in an international health consulting firm specializing in organizational innovation and health service transformation. His career has been characterized by an unflagging commitment to the concepts of shared governance, effective partnership, and the development of the human capacity to understand and manage change. Dr. Porter-O'Grady serves as a corporate director of two of the largest not-for-profit health systems in the country: Franciscan Health Partnerships and Catholic Health East. He has a master's in nursing and business administration, a doctorate in learning behavior, and a doctorate in health systems. He is a certified clinical specialist in gerontology, a registered mediator, and a fellow of the American Academy of Nursing.

Linda L. Roman is president and CEO of HELP Innovations, Inc. Her company created the patented resourceLINK™ telehome health care system that provides skilled nursing visits using two-way interactive television. The company has complete business, marketing, sales, and engineering departments. A respected leader and pioneer in the telehome health care market, Ms. Roman has experience in voluntary association management with the American Cancer Society, in health care product distribution with Procter and Gamble, and as regional manager and administrator of 720 nursing home beds in six locations throughout the Midwest. She holds a bachelor of science degree in health care administration from Wichita State University.

Michael R. Schreurs is president and founder of Schreurs and Associates and Strategic America in Des Moines, serving clients with strategic marketing, planning, and creative execution. His firm's work has been recognized for national innovation and effectiveness in a variety of market segments, including insurance, financial services, entertainment, education, fast food, and governmental services. A graduate of the University of Northern Iowa, Cedar Falls, Mr. Schreurs serves on a number of civic, educational, and corporate boards, providing insight into marketing and business opportunities.

Donnetta Webb, MA, has more than 25 years of experience in education, organization development, and training. She is currently director of network education for Carondelet Health Network in Tucson. Her previous professional experience includes director of corporate training and development, Foundation Health Systems in Sacramento; director of organization development and training, FHP, Phoenix; and regional manager, organization development and training, American Express World Wide Travel Network, Phoenix. Ms. Webb has been a University of Phoenix faculty member since 1983. She has a master's degree in educational psychology and measurements from the University of Nebraska, Lincoln, and is currently engaged in postgraduate work in educational leadership and administration at the University of Arizona. She is an active member of the American Society for Quality, International Society for Performance Improvement, and Phi Delta Kappa.

Foreword

E xpectations for the roles of nurses in executive practice reflect an admixture of futuristic visions of health care and the practical reality of change. This fifth bookazine in the American Organization of Nurse Executives (AONE) Leadership series cuts through this dichotomy by dealing with one of nursing's central issues: its economic base. *Market-Driven Nursing: Developing and Marketing Patient Care Services* is a powerful title because it means that nurse leaders no longer are debating the pros and cons of nursing as a business (the topic of the first bookazine in the series), but are now engaged in the complicated processes of defining nursing services and creating business plans. They are looking at services more comprehensively and identifying the parameters needed to make them whole; that is, of sound clinical quality and adequately financed.

NEW CHALLENGES

The art and science of nurse executive practice have expanded to include new levels of thought and action. The result is a new view of the world, new competencies, and new collaborative relationships. And, of course, there are new challenges. Experiences of changing nursing executive practice shared by AONE members document the fact that nurses currently are leaders in the initiatives to design, facilitate, and manage patient care. Members are sharing how they are managing the complex process of acquiring and configuring resources for services that match both patient demand and need throughout the continuum of care. The challenge of the day is to create new services for which there are few prototypes or even precedents. For example, despite the health promotion and wellness initiatives of the past, fiscally sound, high-quality clinical services for wellness and health are a new "service" challenge in the current health care environment. Another new service challenge revolves around the sense of wholeness in patient care services that includes and accounts for the different needs of varying population groups in service areas.

However, the new challenges to nursing are not just about providing practical wellness services that are supported fiscally; they also are about identifying outcomes that make sense for healthy communities. For example, the process of defining community and patient population groups is a challenge, as is that of designing services that facilitate full patient participation in decision making throughout the care continuum. Another challenge, although not new to nurses in executive practice, is that of appropriately allocating resources to balance service demand with service delivery. And an evolving challenge, not only for nurse executives but also for their colleagues in other fields, is that of defining meaningful outcomes and their indicators.

The complexity of today's practice is reflected in the fact that today's challenges can be classified. There are the typical challenges, such as developing new competencies, but there also are the marathon challenges, such as creating new services, the vocabulary for the new services, and the financing and the structure to make the new services work. The mix and pace of challenges make today's executive practice unique.

Fortunately, nurses in executive practice are not facing the challenges alone. Every member of the executive team is learning. Executive teams now are facing what departments faced in the early days of total quality management. In those days, work focused on tearing down silos that encased departments. These days, work focuses on tearing down the silos that encase the dimensions of service—financial, clinical, public relations, environmental—and those that encase the organization and business structures. The once clear separation between clinical, financial, and administrative dimensions is blurring as executive teams challenge practices to look at new ways of doing business.

Technology will allow a new configuration and integration of all the dimensions of patient care—to shape the new whole of care delivery, including all the dimensions mentioned above. Nurses in executive practice, with their long history and track record for organizing, coordinating, mediating, and innovating, today are challenged to help establish a framework for the whole, to develop valid, reliable service evaluations, and to use the evaluation results effectively to improve patient care. A new wholeness is a characteristic of health care services envisioned in the new millennium.

CONTINUING CHALLENGES

Although much is changing, much remains the same. Health care will continue to be a personal experience, a local service, and a community asset. Because it is local, nurses in executive practice still must know their communities and take steps to ensure that appropriate and relevant services are available to the "whole." As health care services become more holistic and resources continue to be scarce, ethical and moral dilemmas will unfold. Health care executives will continue to have to make quick decisions without the luxury of time to ponder the deeper meanings of their actions. In a perfect world, questions concerning health care as a right and privilege, individual choice, and access to high-quality care should be asked each time services are designed and evaluated.

The most important continuing challenge for nurses in executive practice will be that of defining and improving quality of care in terms that have meaning for patients in the realms of choice, access, and decision-making power. Managing market demand for services has the potential to create a new view of patient services that indeed places the patient in the decision-making position.

The notion of managing market demand for nursing services developed by Judith Ryan, editor of this bookazine, is viewed as a challenge for nurses in executive practice. She has selected content that offers a well-designed journey, taking the reader from a thoughtful analysis of the meaning of nursing care to learning about the process of business planning that integrates it all and ending with a thoughtful discussion of some deep and lasting moral concerns.

Marjorie Beyers, PhD, RN, FAAN
Executive Director
American Organization of Nurse Executives

Preface

About a year ago, I became painfully aware of the subtle, but profound, difference between developing clinical nursing services from the perspectives of professionally determined need and/or regulatory and public policy–driven need and the more direct response to market-driven demand for nursing services. Ed Howell and I were meeting with clinical nursing leadership in our Division of Children's and Women's Services to celebrate success stories in nursing practice. The University of Iowa Hospitals and Clinics (UIHC) had just won the Sigma Theta Tau award for research utilization, and project teams were showcasing innovative applications of AHCPR guidelines for pain management and a unique wellness program that enabled working mothers to breast-feed their babies at the work site.

Ed acknowledged that both pieces of work were good and exciting, appropriately responsive to public policy and nursing research focused on the general health and well-being of the public. Then, comfortable that he was meeting with some of the country's most highly skilled clinical leaders, he asked if we could accept a challenge. We willingly accepted, and he responded as follows: "Public policy no longer drives the funding for your work. The marketplace is now the driver. If you intend to have continued roles in enhancing the general health of the public, somebody, somewhere along the line, has to pay for it. Nothing good happens out of good intent alone; it has to have a funding base. Will the consumer choose a health plan or provider group that offers expertise in pain management as opposed to one that does not? Will a young mother choose to work at the University of Iowa because of access to the opportunity to breast-feed at the work site? Have you built lasting partnerships with physicians, administrators, and marketing staff to ensure that the public perceives and values the advantages these programs offer and [that] the support structure exists to keep them in place? . . . As an academic medical center, we attract and assume risk for patients with complex chronic disease and comorbid conditions. How do your initiatives contribute to this institution's ability to manage tertiary referral activity? How do they align with our strategic intent to reduce risk and improve the overall health of very focused patient populations? How is nursing at the University of Iowa Hospitals and Clinics positioning itself to respond to market-driven reform of health care?"

We were taken aback by Ed's challenge. In fact, as nurses and clinicians, we resented his questions. Patients and families knew we were making a difference. The nursing profession acknowledged our work. We were confident that our practice was evidence based.

But Ed's challenge opened our eyes. Over several months, we developed a common set of assumptions about the future of health care. We reached a consensus that:

- There is an unmet market demand for nursing services.
- The ability to structure mutually supportive partnerships will be key to successful functioning in the future environment.
- The historical role of managed care—buying and directing care on behalf of employers in an attempt to control costs—will be replaced by a competitive market model where focused care systems will compete against each other for increasingly sophisticated purchasers or consumers. These care systems will self-organize around distinct competencies and geographic and patient groups.

We also learned that nursing leadership needs to develop a skill set and apply a set of instruments and tools to manage the market demand for nursing services. And we learned that we could not find those resources in current nursing and health care management texts. So that is what this book is about. Some of the country's most entrepreneurial health care leaders—many of whom are nurses—have come together to provide the basic building blocks for a meaningful, practical strategy for nurse executives to use to respond to the shifting needs for caregiving.

In chapter 1, "Strategic Partnerships for the Future," Tim Porter-O'Grady explores how nurse executives might create and sustain new partnerships within their health care organization, with partners outside their organization, and between and across personal and public health services. In chapter 2, "Model for Defining Unmet Health Needs," Kristine M. Gebbie suggests that unmet health needs present opportunities to make greater progress toward higher levels of health and describes a model for identifying such needs and devising plans to meet them. In a case study at the back of this chapter, Karen Brugler illustrates how an unmet health need was dealt with at Lutheran General Hospital through development of a diagnostic breast center. In chapter 3, "Developing a Winning Business Plan," Mae Taylor Moss describes how to write a business plan that will keep everyone involved in a project—partners, employees, and even subcontractors—clear about the organization's direction and the project's marketability. Added to chapter 3 is a case study provided by Beverly Folkedahl describing a business plan developed by University of Iowa Hospitals and Clinics (UIHC) for the provision of wound, ostomy, and continence services to outside agencies.

In chapter 4, "Business Product Development," Linda L. Roman focuses on the process of creating viable nursing services products. Her chapter is supported by a case study written by Jody Kurtt and Martha Boysen describing development of a practice plan for ARNPs at UIHC. Mae Taylor Moss produced chapter 5, "Financial Resources for Nursing Entrepreneurial Ventures," in which she defines various types of financing sources and identifies different means of raising start-up capital for ventures outside established organizations. The information in that chapter is supported by a case study, "Forging New Partnerships for Financial Development," written by Norma M. Lang and Lois Evans, relating the experience of the University of Pennsylvania School of Nursing in building a model academic nursing practice that integrates clinical services with education and research. In chapter 6, "Marketing for Change," Michael R. Schreurs provides a framework for marketing nursing products and services. In chapter 7, "Performance Management," Mary Anne McCrea, Donnetta Webb, and Gerri S. Lamb explore the application of performance management concepts to nursing practice in today's health care environment. And finally, in chapter 8, "Nurses in the Marketplace: A Moral Option?" Laurence J. O'Connell offers a discussion of morality and ethics in today's market-driven health care system and the advocacy role that nurses can take to ensure the common good.

In today's marketplace, physicians are aggressively learning to manage market demand for medical care. If nurses are to build mutually supportive partnerships with physicians in the future, nurse leaders must accelerate efforts to introduce and differentiate nursing services in the marketplace. We hope this book will give you the tools to move into a future in which patients and families understand, value, and choose to purchase the very powerful combination of nurse and physician services.

Judith A. Ryan, PhD, FAAN
President and CEO
Evangelical Lutheran Good Samaritan Society

with

R. Edward Howell
Director and CEO
University of Iowa Hospitals and Clinics

1

Strategic Partnerships for the Future

Tim Porter-O'Grady, EdD, PhD, FAAN

Transition into a new age and the transformation of health care in America together form the foundation for new roles and approaches in the delivery of nursing services well into the twenty-first century. This chapter focuses on the emerging realities of this new age and the business and service requirements for nursing within the new context. Characteristics of the health system, their impact on nursing, and the changes necessary if the nursing profession is to thrive are explored. Also discussed are new leadership requirements for nurse executives that will help them lead the profession into a new framework for service delivery.

EMERGING REALITIES IN HEALTH CARE

For decades the nursing profession has been struggling to create a unique identity for itself as a discipline and for its members as individual practitioners. Through concerted political and social initiatives, many resulting from the women's movement, nursing has made considerable advancements in achieving the goals of identity and independence and some improvement in equity. While there is still much to do in the area of equity, the progress of the past 50 years has been impressive, and advancements within the profession in academic and scientific relevance have been significant. Nurses have achieved much for which they can be proud in the journey toward full professional status.

In the past two decades, however, sociopolitical, economic, and technological changes have shifted the rules for behavior, relationships, and effectiveness for everyone. Competition today is embedded in a historic pattern of behavior in which groups or individuals achieved success often at the expense of others in an endless round of jockeying,

1

reconfiguring, pressuring, and positioning in an effort to change power relationships and gain the advantage.

A consensus is emerging that puts forward a different theory of success in the information age. The ability to build real, sustainable connections through telecommunications, satellites, fiber-optics, the Internet, and other new technologies has changed the range of social and business imperatives. Systems science teaches us that interface, relatedness, confluence, integration, and aggregation are the real foundations of sustainable value in the future. The race for individual identity and value and the drive for ascendancy and unilateral advancement at the expense of synergy, synthesis, aggregation, and comprehensiveness are no longer viable behaviors that lead toward sustainable opportunities for the future. What does lead to long-term success is interdependence and interaction. Incremental opportunities and advantages can be obtained through unilateral or highly competitive efforts, but truly sustainable outcomes cannot. Increasingly, the future of enterprise will depend on the kinds of relationships that can be built, the fluidity of those relationships, and the degree of interaction that can be created to sustain and advance the system as a whole.

Foundations of Partnership

Partnership is the password for the new millennium. It is imbued with the essentials for creating viability and constructing a preferable future. Yet for many people and organizations, it is a new paradigm and calls for a new range of strategies and behaviors. The challenge will be to move past old patterns of behavior, action, and self-limiting compartmentalism to engage in newer patterns of response. Some of the activities that must be relegated to the wastebasket of history might be:

- Political lobbying for unilateral positioning or advantage when to do so is clearly at the expense of the greater good
- Hiding behind idealistic posturing for opportunities that clearly create disadvantages for others
- Seeking to further refine unilateral identities and roles in order to ensure value with no discernable or sustainable outcome
- Holding onto past practices when there is no need for them any longer because of new technology or changing demand
- Reacting to necessary changes by substituting smoke screens for real response and constructing diversions and synthetic issues that delay or bypass engagement
- Creating enemies in order to cloud the issues

The foundation of real partnership is the necessity of honest engagement and a willingness to embrace the struggles inherent in creating it.

Building partnerships of any kind means confronting past practices that precluded partnering. This calls for a level of personal and organizational honesty and commitment that is hard to find in many health care organizations. It is evident from the literature that most organizations are going into this changing health care environment reluctantly and are meeting the demand for change with many reservations.

Driven predominantly by economic and financial forces, the health care system is being forced to respond in ways that threaten its past configuration. Hospitals see a loss of bed-based services, physicians a reduction of control and revenue, nurses a loss of jobs and influence, consumers fewer choices and less service, and society fewer entitlements and options. What partnerships there are exist as a way of preserving, defending, and positioning for survival rather than to fully engage in creating the future. New ways of providing health care services must be created that are more cost effective than in the past, of higher quality, health-driven, and that encourage good stewardship of the health care enterprise. The partnerships that will last are those that see these new configurations as opportunities to position themselves for a thriving and sustainable future.

Nursing's Partnership with the Health Care Enterprise

Nursing is rarely seen as a business enterprise. However, its future depends on how well it engages the emerging realities in health care and behaves as a mature partner in the unfolding health care enterprise. The current struggle is to establish a legitimate place at the table where the future gets constructed. Never again can nursing be viewed as a compartmental or departmental service.

Factors Essential to Success   The realities of the age call for a thorough understanding of a number of factors essential to future success in health care service:

- The financial parameters for service delivery are becoming more important every day. No health service can thrive without a clear understanding and articulation of its contribution to the financial health of the system.
- Process knowledge is useful but has no sustainable value unless it is directly connected to outcome. Nurses have an inordinate attachment to process, giving less attention to documenting their direct contribution to outcome and sustainable value.
- While the profession has been effective in carving out a place for nurses in service decisions, little effective strategic or political work has been done to position nurses to have a more

direct share in strategic or financial decisions affecting health service delivery.

- Vision has been too narrow to accurately position the profession as a "best buy" option. Instead of increasing the number of professional nurses in the reorganization of clinical services, in the short term most organizations have actually attempted to reduce the number.

Fortunately, the demand for change in health care service delivery has created circumstances that make it impossible for the profession to continue to live in disciplinary isolation. Like any service (business) enterprise, two things will occur in the work of nurses that will advance their viability:

1. A clear notion of nursing-specific service outcomes
2. Documentation of the value of nursing processes in light of their contribution to outcomes and the financial viability of the system

However, this will not be accomplished by the nursing profession alone. Instead, it will be accomplished through the partnerships that nurses build with others who are also committed to adding value to the health system. In health care, the definition of partnership centers around the equitable agreement among key stakeholders to undertake the essential related processes that will move them collectively to a jointly derived outcome for a mutually acceptable return. Inherent in this definition is an understanding that there is no sustainable future without some well-defined notion of quid pro quo.

Business Principles That Apply to Service Provision   All nurses must now recognize and articulate an understanding of good business principles as they apply to good clinical practice. It is not enough for them to know these principles. They must be able to manage and strategize the advancement of patient services in conjunction with other providers for mutual advantage. To achieve sustainability means reading the signposts of the changing times and putting together a concerted response that positions all the stakeholders as real partners in practice. A number of basic rules now apply to all service provision and practice frameworks in health care, such as the following:

- All invested stakeholders having an impact on the outcomes must be a part of the planning from strategy through funding, protocol, and practice. There is no sustainability without ownership.
- Good stewardship requires that all work have value. Any activity or initiative must itemize the attendant costs and price essential to its exercise.

- If an initiative does not reduce cost, advance outcome without advancing cost, or in some way increase margin, then it clearly should not be undertaken.
- Nothing should be done simply because someone suggests it is a good thing to do. A thing is good to do if it respects predefined financial parameters, improves outcomes, and adds value.
- Incorporated into every practitioner's rule is the understanding that every action is subject to the discipline of value, and that nothing can or should be undertaken if it doesn't advance patient outcomes, reduce required inputs over time, and increase the financial viability of the providers.

As systems emerge as the predominant model of organization, everyone who is a member is a stakeholder and has a personal obligation for the success of the enterprise. One of the most significant activities of leadership is making every member of the system aware of this. A successful service structure depends on individual members and is not simply driven by the insight and energy of those at the top of the organization or those coerced into undertaking action.

EMERGING PARTNERSHIPS FOR THE FUTURE

In systems settings, it is important that leaders recognize the seamless continuum of essential task and relationship components necessary to successfully undertake the work of the system, and that trouble in one area of work or practice ultimately leads to trouble in all areas. For example, the distinctions between inpatient and outpatient are becoming less important than are the linkages between them that define the appropriateness, kind, and quality of service that will be provided over the patient's life span. The distinction is today more a measure of intensity than differentiation.

The characteristics of the entrepreneur are now a basic requisite for all providers in the system regardless of their role or position. Following are required behaviors for every practitioner:

- A basic recognition that unilateral, institutional, and compartmental decisions or strategies do not lead to adequate engagement or sustainable outcomes is essential.
- Good relationships must be promulgated among all disciplines, and the work of the time is the building and reinforcing of strong relationships across the continuum of services in the system.
- Transformation brings with it a demand to read the context for change well and early enough to be able to do something about

it, before so much of the future is already defined that people end up having little control over what form it takes.

- Opportunity is only opportunity if it is to the advantage of all parties. A preferable future cannot be sustained if it brings advantage to one partner at the expense of another.
- Partnership makes for strange bedfellows. A partnership is appropriate if it benefits the parties to it and enables them to do better work.
- Entrepreneurial partnerships should exist only for the time that each partner contributes value and advances mutual outcomes; when value is no longer present the purpose of the relationship is gone.

Understanding the basic tenets of entrepreneurship and partnership is essential to the success of service ventures of any kind. Many types of ventures and partnerships will need to be formed over the next two decades in order to create relationships along the health continuum to ensure an effective and viable health system.

Three kinds of essential partnerships will be necessary to ensure that nursing services thrive into the future: partnerships with physicians, partnerships with employers, and partnerships within a setting (intrepreneurial) and between settings (entrepreneurial) in the community.

Partnerships with Physicians

Nurses have a checkered history in their relations with physicians. In the past few decades doctors have been treated as the enemy and engaged in battle. At best, nurses have viewed them as a necessary evil; at worst, as money-driven guests determined to make the lives of nurses more difficult.

The physician, however, is not the natural enemy of the nurse. Political and gender-based difficulties aside, the most natural relationship in health service exists between nurses and physicians. It is time to reestablish that relationship. In fact, the ability of both to thrive is now dependent on their interaction and mutual support.

Managed care has created an environment that requires more integration of services along a continuum and earlier engagement of consumers in the management of their health. Both will be essential to ensure viable, cost-effective, and efficient health services within a capitated environment. Within these challenges exists a host of opportunities for nurses and physicians to work together, including the following:

- Hospital or health system nursing services can meet all the nursing-related service needs of a physician practice and manage them in the context of the physician's own practice.
- Health system clinical information systems could be directly tied to physician offices so all clinical data are available to physicians directly in their own offices, and all nursing staff have direct access to information on every patient and physician on staff.
- All case management, patient referral, and follow-up services can be provided by nurses as a service to physician practices.
- Advanced practice nurse and hospital nurse services can be made available to physician practices as a way of linking and extending clinical services and relationships and assisting physicians in meeting time and service demands.
- Team and group practice arrangements should include a strong relationship between nurses and physicians. Nurses are eminently qualified to coordinate such teams and, in partnership with physicians, manage the interprofessional relationships as well as the patient's progress.
- Staff clinical development services, patient education processes and programs, medical staff education, and clinical team development are all areas of service and support provided by organized nursing service businesses. As the profession becomes more decentralized, with specialization in patient pathways programs, product lines, or other service constructs, education and support services provide a way of linking nurses to each other and to the rest of the medical community.

The more nurses look at nursing as a business service for which there is a value and price, the better the prospect of providing a viable service. Physicians are customers of considerable value to whom nurses have much to offer. New nursing services can increase nursing value, make connections to physicians that are sustainable for both, and advance the financial quid pro quo.

Increasingly, nurses, especially advanced practice nurses, will need to become partners in physician practices. No longer being employees of the physician but partners in the practice will change the relationship between nurse and physician and create an equitable obligation to the practice's success. Dialogue, relationships, and professional dynamics change considerably when the members of a practice are also its owners. This reflects a more fully developed relationship between the disciplines and increases the demand on both to communicate, interact, and contribute in a mature and professional manner. More equity-based and business relationships between nurses and physicians should increase understanding, respect, and the ability to advance the patient's best interests.

Partnerships with Employers

One of the greatest opportunities for nurses in the near future lies in the area of employer health services. There is a strengthening relationship between health services and the employers who pay for health care. As that grows, a new foundation for health is emerging, with accountability expanding to include both the user and the payer of health services.

It is said that the payer is becoming more interested in the health care of subscribers. Employers are coming to understand that there is a strong relationship between engagement in health activities and reduction in cost for health services used by employees. The notion of early-engagement health services creates a demand for a tighter relationship between payer and employer, including provision of on-site services and direct interaction between provider and employer.

Ways to Advance the Nursing-Employer Connection   There are many ways in which the nursing profession can advance the connection with the employer and the management of the health of their workers, including the following:

- On-site clinics where health care is provided within the work environment for all employees
- Early health assessment activities that establish a baseline for potential health service requirements for all workers
- Contracted occupational health services that focus on safety and health issues at the work site affecting the work and the worker
- Interdisciplinary primary and support services for the employer provided on site or at the provider's setting
- Health education for workers as a way of increasing their accountability for and ownership of their own health
- Family support processes that ensure that life management issues are included in health service
- Counseling and mental health services provided on site either through the employer's employee assistance program or a program managed by the preferred provider
- Rehabilitation and exercise services provided to workers on site to ensure maximum health and to meet special needs
- The application of continuous quality assurance processes for measuring and validating service viability and advancing the clinical delivery of valuable service

All of these services can be coordinated and managed by nurses through a variety of approaches either within the payment structure or by contractual arrangements or group practice designs. The business constructs that underpin these service relationships can be managed as easily by nurses as by any other group. Indeed, nurses have an edge because of their focus on the continuum of care and experience with life span services in a wide variety of settings.

Business Skills A direct relationship with the employer will require the development of clinical business skills, an assertive sense of product, and an ability to compete with others who would like to manage the same subscriber base. Some of these business skills include the following:

- An organized approach to describing and presenting service options to interested subscribers or buyers and creation of marketing materials
- Pricing skills that ensure a good service-cost-price relationship and a return on service sufficient to expand, improve service, or advance profitability
- Creation of a strong capital-planning process to gather the financial resources needed to ensure effective service
- Good sales and interpersonal skills to engage the buyer and build the necessary relationships that sustain the contract
- An ability to create strong interdisciplinary programs that build the provider interfaces necessary to sustain a clinical service structure
- A good sense of the market and the competition as a means of testing programs and services in order to remain current or push service and the market to the next level of innovation

It is critical that nurses recognize that services are not attractive to buyers because they are good. There must be a much stronger relationship established between the value of the program and the interests of the buyer. Most businesses exist to make money for their owners and stockholders. For them "good" means anything that advances their profitability, increases productivity, and significantly reduces the cost of doing business. This orientation is sometimes difficult to understand in the context of such a desirable "product" as health. The relationship between the good health of workers and the value and viability of the business must be made clear to the employer. It should never be assumed that any decision will be made regarding health service simply on the basis of the need for good health. Nurse contractors should make the buyer's argument of a beneficial financial impact long before the buyer of service has to ask for it. It is vital for nurses to know that, in business relationships, one must always see the world from the perspective of the payer if a sustainable association is ever to be established.

Partnerships with the Community

Fortunately, policy makers and community leaders are beginning to see health care as a societal issue of sizable proportions. A community mandate to attend to the health of its members will result in an improved quality of life and a reduction in the socially generated costs associated with debilitation and illness.

Move toward Health Prescription Practices   As health is more broadly defined, the interaction among all of the elements that influence health becomes quite complex. Also, health service providers have an increasing sense of responsibility for the communities within which they reside. Accreditors, regulators, and measurers of quality are increasingly attempting to quantify contribution to community as a basic obligation of health service systems.

The effort to focus on preventive health services instead of sickness-driven activities requires health systems to configure mission and values very differently than in the past. The challenge for the provider is to be able to consider the provision of service within a broader context of health. Influencing the onset of sickness are a host of intersecting variables that, left unaddressed, result in increasing levels of social, mental, and physical illnesses and social and financial costs that continue to increase at an untenable rate.

Nurses too must shift their focus from illness-based activities toward health prescriptive practices. The profession has essentially been co-opted by institutional and bed-based activities to the extent that 60 percent or more of nurses practice in bed-related activities. Nursing's origin, however, was firmly grounded in broader social health prescriptions, such as care of the poor and mentally ill, public health, and military care. Each of these in some measure influenced the foundations of scientific nursing practice.

The move to a stronger focus on community health is a call to nurses to return to these roots and build a strong community infrastructure that focuses on community issues and empowers the community to focus on its own health. Although the temptation is to focus on incremental activities that address segments of the community, the goal should be to build a comprehensive and interacting systematic approach to addressing community health that is facilitated and coordinated by nurses.

Opportunities for Building Effective Coalitions and Service Constructs   As more resources are directed toward community programs, it will be important for nurses to be judicious in their stewardship and use of those dollars. Focusing on a range of activities with a broad impact on community health is more effective than simply concentrating on one aspect of service and devoting skill, time, and dollars to it. Some of these initiatives might include the following:

- Parish nurse programs that make the health of the parish community the center of the nursing practice and focus on the responsibility of members of the parish community to each other across the life span
- Community nursing centers in poor, underserved areas, in elder communities, or among specific populations to help these populations become self-directed and to empower them to address their own unique health service needs
- Interdisciplinary service outreach programs from hospitals and health systems specifically designed for designated populations aligned with the service focus of the system (for example, cancer care, women's health, or children's services)
- Continuing education and health awareness programs that reach out to the community, offered in sites and circumstances that make it easy for people to attend
- Health community initiatives that link providers, policy makers, and community activists together in a comprehensive alliance to address complex community health service needs
- Nursing coalitions directed toward providing nursing leadership in the political arena and in public forums where decisions about health care are influenced and/or made

There is an increasing opportunity in each of these areas for nursing leadership to build effective coalitions, service constructs, and lasting partnerships that advance the health of the community.

EMERGING ROLES FOR NURSE EXECUTIVES

Nurse executives have a real opportunity to provide strong leadership in each of the areas of change. The focus of leadership, however, cannot remain hospital based. Institutional nursing service is no longer the frame of reference for the future of nursing practice or leadership. The nurse executive must see herself as the administrative advocate for people in all settings who believe health should be the focus of the work of health service providers. Linking and integrating patient care personnel around this mission is a critical task of the nurse leader no matter where he or she is located in the system.

Each of the opportunities and challenges discussed in this chapter require well-informed and systems-oriented leadership. None of them can unfold or be operationally successful unless they are well conceived, well executed, and evaluated for their contribution and viability. Nurse executives must be prepared to operate in a forum and format far beyond the constructs of the health system in which they began their leadership practice. (See figure 1-1.) Significant shifts in the role of the nurse leader include the following:

- Rather than leading nurses, the nurse executive now leads patient care activities by linking and integrating health providers.
- Strategic activities now take up an increasing amount of the time and work of the nurse executive. Positioning and planning for a broader framework of health services are critical to the viability of the profession.
- Business planning and structuring contractual relationships with businesses and the community are increasingly important. New health service constructs require good business skills and sound service foundations.
- Relationships are the critical variable affecting the future of health care. The nurse executive is a primary player in the formation and building of relationships among disciplines, services, systems, communities, and businesses.
- Making sure that nursing fits into the emerging models of health service in a wide array of settings is an important component of the new leader's success. Pushing the nursing profession into new service areas and constructs will require determination, single-mindedness, and a thick skin.
- The nurse executive seeks and accepts positions on multiple boards of trustees and public boards for both established and emerging organizations, thus assuring a strong service orientation within these entities.

FIGURE 1-1. Functional Role Behavior Shifts

Institutional	Intrapreneurial	Entrepreneurial
Vertical roles	Horizontal roles	Horizontal relationships
Hierarchy	Partnership	Collateral relationships
Compartmentalized projects	Integrated systems	Alliances
Fragmented initiatives	Collaborative efforts	Cohesive action
Linear lines of authority	Equal partnerships	Relational behavior
Fixed thinking	Flexible thinking	Fluid thinking
Responsible to superiors	Accountable to partners	Accountable to customers
Functional focus	Internal focus	Interactional focus

- The nurse executive advocates for appropriate and effective service frameworks and models. This means assuming leadership around viable choices and contesting those preferences that compromise safety, sustainability, and long-term financial viability of the system.
- The nurse executive makes sure that the information infrastructure necessary to advance highly complex and integrated activities is in place, is accessible to users, and produces desirable and viable outcomes.
- The nurse executive recognizes that the differences between public and private initiatives are increasingly artificial. Greater focus on such public/private enterprises as healthy community programs, interagency collaboration, public/private service arrangements, and private contracting for public services will emerge over the next decade.

Clearly, the nurse executive today must exhibit a level of sophistication and competence considerably in advance of previous expectations. The nurse executive is the front person, model maker, integrator, initiator, and leader in a variety of places and positions that advance health service and nursing practice. The newer models of health service and the systems constructs that provide their context necessitate that this leader be capable of operating in complex and highly interactive environments.

CONCLUSION

The world of nursing practice that we all grew up in no longer exists as a construct for service. Integrated systems and multifocal continuums have become the foundation for the health system. As the complexities of this service environment grow and systems emerge to address them, the nurse executive will need to provide leadership in the areas of transformation, business development, and service structuring and provision across a broad spectrum of environments and structures. Visibility, leadership, and the ability to build strong relationships and maintain disparate and sometimes desperate interactions across the service continuum will be essential talents in this environment. Facilitating diversity among people and systems will be the keystone of the skill sets necessary to ensure success in the role and sustainability in the health care system.

Clearly, it is a time of great excitement and challenge for every practitioner and leader in health care. No one's role is left untouched by the drama affecting the reconfiguration of health services today. It is in these times that the quality and depth of leadership are tested. In the fire of this transformation, the role of the nurse leader is to take on the challenge to be a more creative, innovative, and contributing member to the health system of the future. Building a preferred future is the primary work of any generation. Ensuring that the future of health care is better than at our point of entry is both the challenge and the work of the time.

Bibliography

American Nurses Association (and 42 Endorsers). *Nursing's Agenda for Health Care Reform* (Washington, DC: American Nurses Association, 1991).

Anderson, Terry. *Transforming Leadership* (Boca Raton, FL: St Lucie Press, 1997).

Andrews, Heather, Lynn Cook, Janet Davidson, Don Schurman, Eric Taylor, and Ronald Wensel. *Organizational Transformation in Health Care: A Work in Progress* (San Francisco: Jossey-Bass Publishers, 1994).

Beckham, Daniel. The Power of Primary Care, *Healthcare Forum Journal* 37, no. 1 (1994): 68–74.

Bostrum, Janet. Impact of Physician Practice on Nursing Care, *Nursing Economic$* 12, no. 5 (1994): 250–55.

Brown, Montague. The Economic Era: Now to the Real Change, *Health Care Management Review* 19, no. 4 (1995): 73–82.

Burda, David. Learn From Fallen Leaders: Don't Neglect Your Constituency, *Modern Healthcare* 21, no. 4 (1991): 24.

Channon, Jim. Social Architecture: Can We Design a New Civilization?, *World Business Academy Perspectives* 9, no. 3 (1995): 19–32.

Drucker, Peter. *The Organization of the Future* (San Francisco: Jossey-Bass Publishers, 1997).

Fagin, Claire. Collaboration Between Nurses and Physicians: No Longer a Choice, *Nursing & Health Care* 13, no. 7 (1992): 354–63.

Frank, Robert, and Philip Cook. *The Winner-Take-All Society* (New York: The Fress Press, 1995).

Heskett, James, Earl Sasser, and Leonard Schlesinger. *The Service-Profit Chain* (New York: The Free Press, 1997).

Kaluzny, Arnold, Howard Zuckerman, and Thomas Ricketts. *Partners for the Dance: Forming Strategic Alliances in Health Care* (Chicago: Health Administration Press, 1995).

Lassen, April, Donna Fosbinde, Stephen Minton, and Mureno Robins. Nurse/Physician Collaborative Practice: Improving Health Care Quality While Decreasing Cost, *Nursing Economic$* 15, no. 2 (1997): 87–91.

Lipman-Blumen, Jean. *The Connective Edge: Leading in an Interdependent World* (San Francisco: Jossey-Bass Publishers, 1996).

Porter-O'Grady, Tim. Building Partnerships in Health Care: Creating Whole Systems Change, *Nursing & Health Care* 15, no. 1 (1994): 34–38.

_____. Shifting Tides: The New Role of the Nurse Executive, *Aspen's Advisor for the Nurse Executive* 10, no. 8 (1995): 1–4.

Ulrich, Beth. *Leadership and Management According to Florence Nightingale* (Norwalk, CT: Appleton & Lang Publishers, 1992).

Wheatley, Margaret. *Leadership and the New Science* (San Francisco: Berrett-Koehler Publishers, 1992).

Woollard, Robert. Choices for a Sustainable Future, *Healthcare Forum* 37, no. 3 (1994): 30–34.

2

Model for Defining Unmet Health Needs

Kristine M. Gebbie, DrPH, RN

M any executives have achieved success by virtue of their ability to redefine problems as opportunities and challenges. Whether changing the boundaries of the resources to be invested, reconsidering the goals and time frames, or discovering/rediscovering possible techniques, it is the continual process of taking in information, defining direction, taking planned action, and assessing progress that are the hallmarks of achievement in any field. In considering the health status of a community or the nation, it is all too easy to focus on the problems: premature mortality from tobacco-related diseases, unintended injuries, rates of adolescent pregnancy and sexually transmitted diseases, or the number of individuals and families lacking a health care "home" or the way to pay for it. Yet for each of these perceived problems, there are examples of communities, agencies, and individuals who have re-cast their thinking, engaged new partners, and made measurable progress toward a higher level of health care.

Unmet health needs are opportunities for nurse leaders to use the redefining process described above to ensure that ways of meeting them are initiated and potential resources identified. They can build coalitions and organizations that move individuals and communities toward higher levels of health. Recognition of unmet needs might come through several sources, such as a personal experience in which needed care was not available, a family encounter with an unresponsive system, a patient admitted for treatment who is far sicker than warranted because of lack of information or access, a local paper's feature article on bicycle/automobile traffic encounters, or an employer threatening to close an unprofitable clinical service. In each case, an individual response may well be warranted, but each case also presents an occasion for seeking a wider definition of the unmet need and making plans for active intervention.

This chapter presents a model for community health improvement planning. It describes a process that a community can use to identify important unmet needs and make plans to meet them. It also discusses how nurses seeking new opportunities might initiate and lead the process. The case study at the back of the chapter describes how nursing contributed to development of a diagnostic breast center in response to a recognized need.

IMPROVING HEALTH IN COMMUNITIES

The Institute of Medicine (IOM) Committee on Using Performance Monitoring to Improve Community Health has developed a model for community health improvement planning that is a useful template for defining unmet (and even unrecognized) needs.* The panel was formed in 1995 in response to the growing interest in performance monitoring as a mechanism for tracking the progress of communities toward public health goals. The committee was asked to "examine how a performance monitoring system could be used to improve the public's health by identifying the range of actors that can affect community health, monitoring the extent to which their actions make a constructive contribution to the health of the community, and promoting policy development and collaboration between public and private sector entities."[1]

In working to fulfill this charge, the committee found that there were many examples of communities achieving health improvement, many of them beginning with identification of unmet needs. But it also found that there was no clearly articulated model of how communities could use information effectively in the process of identifying needs, selecting which should receive priority for intervention, developing plans of action, and holding participants accountable for their share of the planned effort.

The panel conducted workshop sessions with participants of exemplary state and local programs, examined available literature on health improvement processes, and considered available health data and various community structures. In its final work, the committee used as a foundation for its model the Evans and Stoddard Field Model of Health,[2] which clearly illustrates that understanding how health is achieved necessitates going far beyond the traditional health system with its linear diagnostic and treatment process. The committee then developed its own model, called Community Health Improvement Process, through which a community can assemble information in order to define directions for action

---

*The committee was co-chaired by Bobbie Berkowitz, PhD, RN, then deputy secretary, Washington State Department of Health, and Thomas Inui, MD, professor and chair, ambulatory care and prevention, Harvard Medical School. The author served on this committee as a liaison from the Institute of Medicine Board on Health Promotion and Disease Prevention.

and move responsibly toward a higher level of health. First, however, a closer look a the Field Model of Health would be helpful.

Field Model of Health

The model advanced by Evans and Stoddard is based on the following tenets:

- Thinking of health as the mere absence of diagnosable disease is inadequate.
- Social and physical environments have a strong influence on individuals.
- Functional status and a sense of well-being are the desirable outcomes of interest.

In figure 2-1, the genetic endowment of the individual is shown on the same line as the social and physical environments, illustrating the complex interaction of external contexts with biological heritage. An individual has a unique pattern of behavioral and biological responses to these factors that develop over a lifetime. Disease is shown as a product of the environment (all aspects) and individual response, modified by available health care. The level of health and function resulting from the combination of individual responses and disease leads to the states of well-being and prosperity (or lack thereof) experienced by the individual. Imagining a bio-psycho-social nursing model and a family- and community-oriented intervention model superimposed over this approach illustrates the way many nurses approach their patients.

This model is useful for considering unmet needs because of the breadth of focus it invites. At the level of the individual patient, it pushes one to think not only of appropriate management of diet and medication schedules, but also whether or not the individual lives in a neighborhood that has accessible pharmacy and grocery services or whether a history of risk-taking behavior will jeopardize long-term management of chronic disease. On the family level, the model encourages taking into account the intertwined behavior patterns of all family members as well as the individual patient's, and understanding that prosperity is directly linked to the process of well-being. Finally, at the community level, the model suggests that those interested in healthier outcomes in the community ought to invite not only the known health partners (hospitals, care systems, and payers) to become involved in community health initiatives, but also those responsible for the physical and social environments (housing, transportation, and environmental protection agencies).

Efforts by nurses to involve family members in a patient's care from the time of hospital admission reflect this broad understanding, as do

FIGURE 2-1. A Field Model of Health

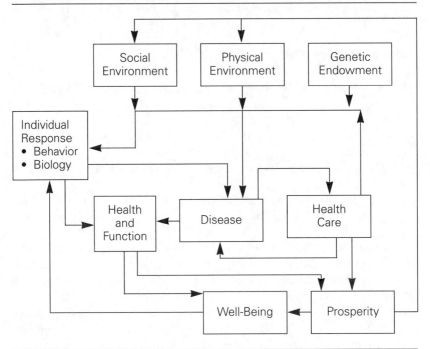

Reprinted from *Social Science and Medicine* 31, R. G. Evans and G. L. Stoddart, Producing Health, Consuming Health Care, p. 1359; copyright 1990, with permission from Elsevier Science.

nurses who engage community members in advocating a lead paint removal project after identifying several toddlers with elevated blood lead levels. Transcultural and cross-cultural nursing efforts share with this model an understanding that the different social experiences of those from different cultural, ethnic, or racial backgrounds will lead to different responses to the same threat to health, and they will need different interventions to restore or maintain a sense of well-being.

This model can facilitate framing health system planning questions to focus attention not only on the illness/health care dyad but on the full spectrum of components necessary to achieve well-being. Unmet needs are often unidentified needs. The need for trauma care or emergency transportation may be unmet in a locality, but it is unlikely that the need would be unknown. One or two incidents in which victims of a traffic crash have to wait hours for a vehicle to move them to an emergency room, or, on arrival at the hospital, they receive inadequate or inappropriate treatment, will make this need evident. On the other hand, unless there is a wide assessment of trauma and injury from a perspective such as the field model, the same community might not identify opportunities to prevent the traffic crash altogether through changing the environment (separating cars and bicycles on the roadway) or changing behavior (initiating a school bicycle safety program).

Community Health Improvement Process

Having determined that a broad understanding of health and its determinants in the community is the appropriate perspective, the IOM committee proceeded to describe a process that could be used by a community to identify high-priority unmet needs and make plans to meet them. This model, the Community Health Improvement Process, is illustrated in figure 2-2. It is a two-level process. The first cycle is at the communitywide, general health status level and is focused on identifying the most important health challenges to which attention should be given. The second level is a series of cycles, one for each of several selected problem areas.

Problem Identification and Prioritization Cycle   The first level of the Community Health Improvement Process is the cycle of problem identification and prioritization. It can begin with a broad health coalition or partnership formed out of a general interest in health improvement that then proceeds to gather data and set priorities. Alternatively, it can begin with a limited number of participants preparing and presenting a community health profile, using the results to interest others in forming a coalition that can then set priorities. In either case, the information to be gathered should be consistent with the field model[3] and include data on:

- Sociodemographic characteristics
- Health status
- Health risk factors
- Health care resource consumption
- Functional status
- Quality of life

Figure 2-3 gives the complete list of suggested data elements in each of these categories.

When the community of interest is a relatively large geopolitical area, it may be difficult to obtain all of the suggested data elements in a timely manner at a reasonable cost. For very small areas, the problem of drawing statistical conclusions based on small numbers becomes critical. What is most important is that those interested in identifying health problems for the community begin with a relatively wide range of information that reflects the full context of health status and the circumstances that might have an affect on health. The particular indicators in figure 2-3 were

FIGURE 2-2.   The Community Health Improvement Process

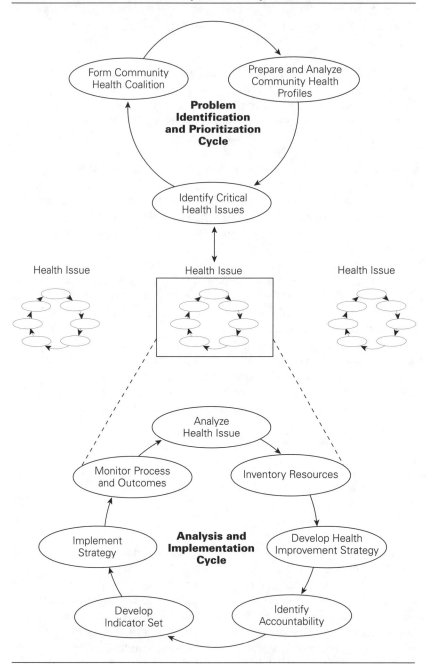

Reprinted, with permission, from J. Durch, L. Bailey, and M. Soto, eds., *Improving Health in the Community: A Role for Performance Monitoring.* Copyright 1997 by the National Academy of Sciences. Courtesy of the National Academy Press, Washington, DC.

FIGURE 2-3. Community Health Profile Indicators

Sociodemographic Characteristics

- Distribution of the population by age and race/ethnicity
- Number/proportion of persons in groups such as migrants, homeless, or non-English-speaking for whom access to services may be a concern
- Number/proportion of persons age 25 and older with less than high school education
- Ratio of the number of graduating (high school) students to number entering ninth grade three years earlier
- Median household income
- Proportion of children under 15 living in families at or below the poverty level
- Unemployment rate
- Number/proportion of single-parent families
- Number/proportion of persons without health insurance

Health Status

- Infant mortality rate by race/ethnicity
- Numbers of deaths or age-adjusted death rate for motor vehicle crashes, work-related injuries, suicide, homicide, lung cancer, breast cancer, cardio-vascular disease, and all causes (by age, race, and gender as appropriate)
- Reported incidence of AIDS, measles, tuberculosis, and primary and secondary syphilis (by age, race, and gender as appropriate)
- Births to adolescents (10–17) as a proportion of total live births
- Number and rate of confirmed abuse and neglect cases among children

Health Risk Factors

- Proportion of 2-year-olds who have received all age-appropriate vaccines
- Proportion of adults age 65 and older who have been immunized for pneu-mococcal pneumonia; proportion immunized in the past 12 months for influenza
- Proportion of the population who smoke (by age, race, and gender as appropriate)
- Proportion of the population age 18 and older who are obese
- Number and type of U.S. Environmental Protection Agency air quality stan-dards not met
- Proportion of assessed river, lakes, and estuaries that support beneficial uses

Health Care Resource Consumption

- Per capita health care spending for Medicare beneficiaries

Functional Status

- Proportion of adults reporting that their general health is good to excellent
- Average number of days in past 30 for which adults report their physical and mental health was not good

Quality of Life

- Proportion of adults satisfied with the health care system in the community
- Proportion of persons satisfied with the quality of life in the community

Reprinted, with permission, from J. Durch, L. Bailey, and M. Soto, eds., *Improving Health in the Community: A Role for Performance Monitoring.* Copyright 1997 by the National Academy of Sciences. Courtesy of the National Academy Press, Washington, DC.

chosen because of their general utility and availability. There may be special populations of interest or some previously suspected health problem not included in the suggested data set that any one community may want to include. When a suggested data element is not available, an effort should be made to substitute some other information of a similar nature or make a best estimate from national or state-level findings.

The result of this first cycle should be the selection of a small number of issues for more detailed analysis and action. The exact number will vary from place to place, depending on the level of concern about the unmet needs, potential priorities suggested by the overview, and the level of resources available to manage and carry out the process. One effect of the broader overview is to put various possible areas of interest into perspective: what may have seemed critical to an uninformed audience fades as the overview reveals previously unidentified areas of high mortality or disparity in access or services between gender or ethnic groups. To the extent feasible, some approach to communitywide involvement in priority setting is appropriate at this point. As platforms for this effort, communities may use the annual planning cycle of the local board of health, a Healthy Communities coalition,[4] the health committee of the local United Way, or a state health agency request for input on setting state health priorities.

A critical part of the effort is an attempt to bring to the table, not only the "usual cast of characters," but also those representative of community groups not previously engaged, especially if they represent a potential area of intervention (a fair housing coalition) or a population at high risk (such as a cluster of newly arrived immigrants).

Analysis and Implementation Cycle   Having selected a small number of issues on which to focus, the analysis and implementation cycle can begin. For each of the health issues selected, the process includes:

- *Analysis of the health issue*—collection of additional, more detailed information in each of the health field model areas as they apply to the problem in question
- *Inventory of resources*—identification of the health professionals and services, government agencies, advocacy groups, and state or national resources that might become a part of a solution
- *Development of a health improvement strategy*—negotiation of an action plan that puts identified resources to work on as many aspects of the problem area as possible, with attention to timing and coordination of effort
- *Identification of accountability*—specific acceptance of responsibility for portions of the strategy by various players, with a setting and timetable for reporting to one another on progress or roadblocks encountered

- *Development of an indicator set*—agreement on what data elements, and what target figure, will be used to measure the accountable parties' progress toward selected goals
- *Implementation*—carrying out the selected action plan
- *Monitoring of implementation and outcomes*—regular feedback loops regarding change in selected indicators and the experience of involved parties

The analysis of any one issue should mimic the overall community analysis done in the first level of the process; that is, it should include gathering and interpreting data relevant to the full scope of the field model of health (listed in figure 2-3), related as specifically as possible to the health problem of interest. The field model, with its wide range of indicators, will push communities to consider whether reduction of a particular health problem would best be accomplished using traditional health resources or whether there are more important unmet needs in the associated physical and social environment or related to existing human behavior patterns. Knowledgeable health professionals, including nurses, are invaluable at this point, as they can highlight known relationships; for example, those between a mother's education level or income and pregnancy outcomes.

A Continuous Process   The IOM report provides detailed discussion of prototypical data sets for nine examples, including breast and cervical cancers, depression, infant health, and violence.[5] However, it is important to point out that the Community Health Improvement Process does not automatically reveal either the most important intervention steps or the most effective way of taking those steps. The expertise of all involved members of the community, including health (and other) professionals; searches of the literature for best practices implemented elsewhere; and community preferences will all enter into the selection of preferred action steps. What distinguishes this process from many others that have appeared in the literature is its assertion that the process is a continuous cycle, from problem identification and prioritization, through implementation and monitoring of outcomes, to a reassessment of the problem and a new action plan, perhaps at annual intervals. The assignment of accountability for specific measures limits the chance that the process will stall as participants encounter difficulty or are drawn to other efforts.

At each cycle, changes in the community may reveal new areas for action and opportunities to shift resources to more promising activities. Further, it is recommended that at some longer time interval, perhaps three to five years, the full community assessment be repeated in order to identify whether new, previously unaddressed health issues have become a problem, and new issue-specific planning and implementation cycles should be begun and old ones closed or moved to a lower priority.

LEADING AND PARTNERING IN THE PROCESS

Adopting the Community Health Improvement Process offers the community a number of advantages, including the following:

- It provides a data-grounded perspective on priorities. Far too many community efforts are undertaken in response to a single attention-getting event without consideration of their relative importance to health.
- It requires the health community to engage in discussion with those having other interests, either in data collection, data interpretation, or program implementation. This minimizes the single-institution crusade experienced in many settings.
- It sets time frames for regular reassessment of activities and encourages a strategic view of investments. This is important if planning participants are to remain involved through implementation and evaluation.
- It specifically supports assignment of responsibility and accountability in what is otherwise a very diffuse process.
- It facilitates the identification of unmet needs by its insistence on a broad look at health and its determinants, whether at the communitywide general health level or within any one area of health concern.

In initiating the health improvement process, two elements must be defined: what constitutes a community and what the various leadership roles within the process will be.

Defining Community

Any community or subset of a community might initiate a Community Health Improvement Process for its members. However, the very definition of community is a challenge. Historically, it has had a narrow geopolitical definition; that is, individuals with a common culture and language in a bounded geographic area living under a common system of governance.[6] Public health departments, tied as they are to geopolitical boundaries, have a responsibility to ensure that all who fall within the assigned area are considered in any planning for improved health. Working with the geopolitical definition of community can mean easier access to usable data sets and a higher level of assurance that often-neglected groups such as the uninsured or racial/ethnic minorities will not be left out of the process. However, the IOM committee took as its definition of community that offered by Labonte: "Individuals with shared affinity, and perhaps a shared geography, who organize around an issue, with collective discussion, decision making and action."[7]

This broader approach is very useful in planning the future direction of a health care system. The mobility of our population, the blurring of daily life across many traditional geopolitical boundaries, and the confluence of community and market interests on the part of many health service provider organizations make it likely that at least some health improvement efforts will focus on community defined in this nongeographic manner. Insurance companies and health maintenance organizations are connected to enrollees. Individual care givers are responsible to those who walk, roll, or are carried into the office, clinic, or hospital. Certainly there is a relationship to the broader circle of people or geography beyond those now connected to the system: as potential future markets, as potential disrupters of ongoing efforts, or as competitors.

The broader approach to defining community allows for the emergence of communities of affinity around issues of common concern that may cross traditional geographic boundaries. Unless they are developed with an overt or covert intent to discriminate, there is no reason such emergent communities cannot effectively complete health assessments and health improvement plans. It is also quite possible that if such a community approaches its task within the frame of the field model of health, it will expand its frame of reference to include some of those parties originally seen as outside the community either because they share the experience of the unmet need or because they can contribute to the preferred solution.

It is appropriate for those involved in a community health improvement process to be reminded of the overall vision of public health: healthy people in healthy communities.[8] If attention is given only to individuals (such as those presenting as patients or clients) and not to the full set of those groups and individuals composing the community within which they work, live, and play, it will not be possible to realize this vision.

Identifying Leadership and Partnership Roles

The possible leadership roles within the health improvement process are many, including:

- Community-level leadership (however the community is defined) to decide to perform the initial communitywide problem identification cycle (Someone has to call the first meeting.)
- Leadership within and across subsets of the community to bring all potentially interested parties to the table to consider what is known about the community and what problems (previously known or not and still unmet) should receive priority attention
- Leadership to approach information gathering and display in a way that is true to the broad model of health and its determinants presented in this chapter

- Leadership to continuously hold people and organizations accountable across the multiyear process

There are similar opportunities for leadership within each problem-specific analysis and implementation cycle. Someone must be the focal point for all efforts on any selected area of action. Leadership will be required once again to:

- Reach broadly into the community to gather the full array of information needed to understand the issue, select action steps, and monitor progress toward goals
- Hold organizations or individuals accountable for the actions they commit to undertake as a part of the implementation cycle
- Deal with the process and politics of reallocating resources during the process (a likely outcome)
- Help those who committed to a specific priority area recognize when it is time to move on to another communitywide analysis and consider moving efforts to some different, newly identified area of unmet need

Just as there are many opportunities for leadership within this process, there are many opportunities for partnership. The broad model of health and the community health improvement process illustrate in many ways the interrelationships of organizations and people with regard to health. No matter how committed and interested any one organization is, and no matter how effective its leaders, it cannot successfully develop a community health improvement process alone. A "command and control" model might be successful in gathering sufficient information about a community to present the initial overview data set. But any effort to select priorities, or to assign responsibility and accountability within a specific priority issue, will be a failure if the others involved do not feel a sense of partnership and ownership. The history of health planning efforts in the United States is replete with plans for which no legacy of implementation or change exists. And the Healthy Communities effort now gaining strength across the country is evidence that partnering works.[9]

THE NURSING ROLE

The cycle of gathering information, making an analytic determination about the meaning of the information and potential for change, selecting action steps, implementing them, and then evaluating the results before once again gathering information and analyzing it preparatory to planning action is remarkably similar to the nursing process as it is usually described. This is definitely an advantage for a nurse encountering the community health improvement process. Another advantage is that the attention to context and forces beyond the biological diagnosis of disease is also familiar. And at least as a principle (though it does get lost in practice), the use of a careful assessment to identify previously unlabeled and thus unmet health needs is one of the priorities in nursing.

Translating all of this to the role of the nurse executive, it is possible to apply a broad model of determinants of health and a community health improvement process within any organizational context. As a health organization considers reconfiguring its services because of economic shifts or anticipated demographic changes, nurse leaders are in a position to gather a much wider range of information than only service-use statistics from a single agency and to put that information into a community context. From such an analysis, any number of previously unrecognized and unmet needs are likely to emerge.

Further, in order to assemble the full range of information suggested by the model and to present it effectively to illustrate the emerging evidence of unmet needs, partnerships with a wide range of individuals, agencies, and community groups will be needed. This assessment and fact-gathering phase can be an effective base for later advocacy that nursing be involved in developing the services and programs that would fill the identified, previously unmet needs.

There are numerous examples of nurses taking entrepreneurial advantage of changes in the health system, such as the neonatal intensive care nurses who began home care services, allowing their tiny charges to be cared for at home far sooner in life and at lower cost. Many more opportunities such as this could be created, some of them within systems and others in the community, with application of a more systematic approach to the process of defining the unmet needs and identifying the possible participants in solutions.

CONCLUSION

Nursing has a strong history of responding to unmet need, from Florence Nightingale in the Crimea, to the creation of organizations such as the Frontier Nursing Service, to today's nurse-owned and -managed long-term care and quality assurance companies. The Community Health Improvement Process, grounded in the field model of health, provides one useful approach for identifying a wide range of unmet needs and stimulating activities to meet them. Nurses in active partnership and leadership in the process will be accepting the challenge of turning problems into opportunities. The potential for a positive impact on health is immense.

References

1. J. Durch, L. Bailey, and M. Stoto. *Improving Health in the Community: A Role for Performance Monitoring* (Washington, DC: National Academy Press, 1997), p. vi.

2. R. G. Evans and G. L. Stoddard. Producing Health, Consuming Health Care, *Social Science and Medicine* 31 (1990): 1359.

3. Durch, Bailey, and Stoto, pp. 129–30.

4. B. C. Flynn. Toward Worldwide Health Promotion, *Annual Review of Public Health* 17 (1996): 299–309.

5. Durch, Bailey, and Stoto, pp. 183–359.

6. K. Gebbie. You, Me, or Us: Prevention and Health Promotion, *American Journal of Preventive Medicine* 9 (1993): 3.

7. R. Labonte. Health Promotion: From Concepts to Strategies, *Health Care Management Forum* 1, no. 3 (1988): 24–30.

8. Public Health Functions Steering Committee. *Public Health in America* (Washington, DC: U.S. Department of Health and Human Services Office of Disease Prevention and Health Promotion, 1994).

9. Flynn.

CASE STUDY: DEVELOPING A DIAGNOSTIC BREAST CENTER

Karen Brugler, MM, LCSW

A prominent trend in health care for the next 30 years is the aging of the population. The issues of middle age for women have already become topics of public interest. Among those issues is the prevalence of breast cancer.

One in eight women will have breast cancer some time in her life. Aware of this statistic, more women are scheduling regular mammography examinations. Because of this increase and because the exams are now capable of spotting smaller lesions, breast biopsies are becoming more common. Medical centers that perform breast biopsies generally have a low rate of positives, so most women who wait for biopsy results have a benign diagnosis.

The turnaround time from identification of a mass or mammographic abnormality to definitive diagnosis is three to six weeks in most health care systems. At Lutheran General Hospital in Park Ridge, Illinois, the goal of the founders of its Diagnostic Breast Center was the reduction of "sleepless nights" for patients awaiting a diagnosis. A unique perspective of nursing in partnership with physicians and hospital administrators was integral to the design of the center.

This case study describes how the Diagnostic Breast Center was developed as a result of the nursing perspective responding and contributing to an unmet societal need.

Creation of the Clinical Guideline for Diagnosis of Breast Problems

Interest in developing a diagnostic breast center for patients of Lutheran General Hospital began in 1992, originating in the Lutheran General Health Plan Medical Directors Group. That group determined that diagnosis of breast disease was the number one reason women visit physician offices. The team serving on the project included physicians from family practice, oncology, radiology, OB/GYN, internal medicine, and general surgery.

The objective of the project was to create a clinical practice guideline to be used by physicians that would reduce the turnaround time from recognition of a breast problem, including identification of a palpable mass or mammographic abnormality, to communication to the patient of a definitive diagnosis. Lutheran General used an internally developed road map as a guide in the algorithm development. (See figure 2-4.)

Guidelines developed by the Institute for Clinical Systems Integration at Park Nicollet in Minneapolis were used as a template or "seed"

FIGURE 2-4.   Road Map for Development of Clinical Algorithms

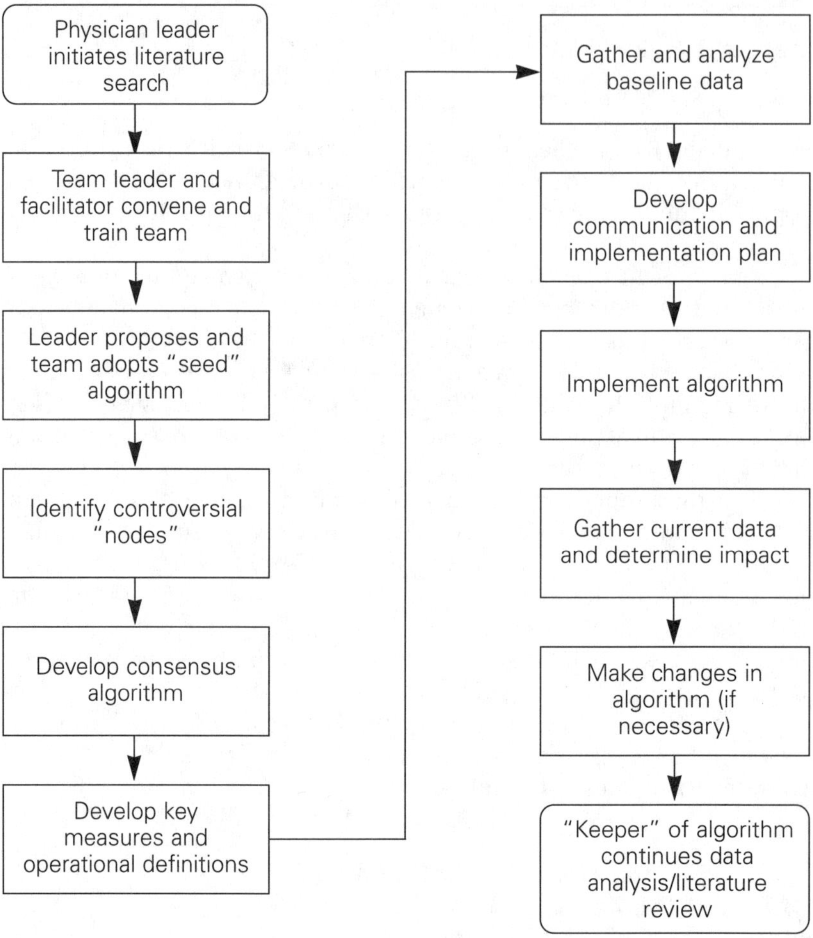

Published with permission of Advocate Health and Hospital Corporation, Oak Brook, IL.

algorithm. When the team members had completed their work, they had developed consensus algorithms for diagnosis of palpable mass and mammographic abnormality. Issues related to the appropriate diagnostic procedure to be used were resolved after many discussions between the physician representatives from radiology and surgery. A measurement plan was put into place that included measures of algorithm compliance, turnaround time, cost, and clinical outcome. (See table 2-1.)

The major focus of implementation of the algorithms was physician education. Physicians from all specialties were educated, and referral forms and internal mechanisms were developed to support compliance with the algorithm. Despite these efforts, the turnaround

TABLE 2-1. Diagnosis of Breast Mass: Data Measurement Plan

Key Concept	Specific Measures	Operational Definitions	Data Source(s)	Collection Method/Schedule
Algorithm Compliance	For patients with procedures: • biopsies • cyst aspirations	• Pre-menopausal patient examined first 10 days of cycle • Patient has breast examination by PCP • Patient had a 6-month f/u mammogram after a negative biopsy	Lutheran General Health Plan (LGHP) identified patients Charts LGHP information systems	6 months Pull all LGHP charts with identified CPT codes LGHP quality improvement staff, radiology, pathology, cancer registry, surgery
Turnaround Time		Time between identification of palpable mass or mammographic abnormality and communication of definitive diagnosis	LGHP patient charts with ICD-9/CPT codes of cyst aspiration, biopsy, and breast mass	6 months
Cost	Costs of: • Surgical referrals • Mammograms • Cyst aspirations • Stereotactic core biopsy • Needle localization procedure	• Total cost of procedure: (mammograms, cyst aspirations, etc.)/number of ICD-9 patients coded with breast mass • Total cost of procedure/number of females greater than 20 years in LGHP • Patients with ICD-9 code breast mass in LGHP/number of females greater than 20 years in LGHP	LGHP information systems	6 months
Patient Outcome	Percent of patients with breast cancer detected in early stages	Number and percent of following: Cancer detected in stages 0–4	Identify LGHP patients with cancer diagnosis Cross-reference with data in cancer registry	6 months Cancer Registry

Published with permission of Advocate Health and Hospital Corporation, Oak Brook, IL.

33

time for diagnosis of breast disease was not improved. Patients continued to wait three to six weeks to be informed of their diagnosis. Clearly,
the development of a clinical practice guideline, although a necessary
first step, did not resolve the process problem of turnaround time.
Process problems require the development of new systems of care that
go beyond the development of clinical practice guidelines to creation of
new roles focused on coordination of care. The role of nursing is particularly well suited to the task of coordination.

Diagnosis of Breast Problems Revisited

Concern about the diagnosis of breast disease surfaced again at Lutheran
General Hospital in 1996, raised by both primary care physicians and
patients, some of whom were employees of the hospital. The current
system of care required the patient to find the right physician, schedule
the right procedure, manage insurance and reimbursement issues,
obtain consensus from the group of doctors responsible for her care,
and decide what action to take in the event of a positive or benign diagnosis. All of this was required of an anxious patient who had to wait for
weeks to put closure on the experience. A more comprehensive intervention was required to address the service issues faced by patients.

In June 1997, at the request of the chief executive of Lutheran General Hospital, a steering committee was formed to consider the development of a comprehensive breast center for members of the Lutheran
General Hospital community. Executive sponsorship was required
because an intervention designed to improve the level of service and
reduce turnaround time required the approval of capital, creation of
new positions, and renovation of space. The scope of the project
changed from developing a "best practice" clinical guideline to providing a newly designed system of care. The chief nursing officer of
Lutheran General was instrumental in defining the center as part of the
hospital strategic plan and framing the structure of the initiative.

The breast center project at Lutheran General had three phases:
sponsorship, development, and implementation. Each of these phases
had its unique challenges.

Sponsorship Phase   The sponsorship phase involved developing a
vision of the breast center and creating an internal mandate to implement it. Before the steering committee convened, a telephone survey
was conducted by an outside consultant with a group of 25 primary care
physicians in family practice, internal medicine, and OB/GYN. These
physicians were asked where they referred patients for mammograms,
key factors in their referral choices, level of satisfaction with mammography services, desired process for follow-up of test results, and interest in a diagnostic breast center. Their responses were used as key

quality characteristics in the subsequent design of the center and included the following suggestions:

- Services to be offered at the center should include physician exam, diagnostic mammography, needle localization biopsy, ultrasound, core biopsies (stereotactic, ultrasound guided, palpable mass), patient education, second-opinion program, and self-referral.
- Equipment in the center should include two mammography units, an ultrasound unit, and a stereotactic core biopsy unit. Location of this equipment in a single space would reduce the number of trips the patient would need to make, providing a "one-stop" diagnostic center.
- Space requirements included office space for a coordinator, a waiting area, a consult/reading room, a dark room, a room designated for education of residents, two mammography rooms with ultrasound, a core biopsy room, and storage space for medical records and films. The physical layout was developed using the list of services to be provided in the center and the type of personnel needed to perform those services.
- Hours should be convenient.
- The center should have a surgeon assigned for each day and available during the hours the center is open, a dedicated radiologist, a scheduler, mammographers, a medical director, and a clinical coordinator.

A draft of the vision statement for the center was developed by the steering committee. It included the following:

- Decrease the time to definitive diagnosis from several weeks to less than one week.
- Utilize clinical guidelines established by a multidisciplinary group of physicians as templates for development of operational processes.
- Provide consultation with a radiologist, including diagnostic mammography, ultrasound, and stereotactic biopsy, during hours the center is open.
- Make immediate consultation with a surgeon available to the patient during hours the center is open. A surgical exam should be provided for all patients referred to the center as designated by the clinical practice guidelines for palpable mass, mammographic abnormality, and nipple problem. (Figure 2-5 reflects that the surgical exam is done for all patients after intake and prior to subsequent diagnostic mammography.)
- Patient education, a second opinion program, and a clinical coordinator should be available to patients for questions or concerns during the process of diagnosis.

FIGURE 2-5. Algorithm for Palpable Mass

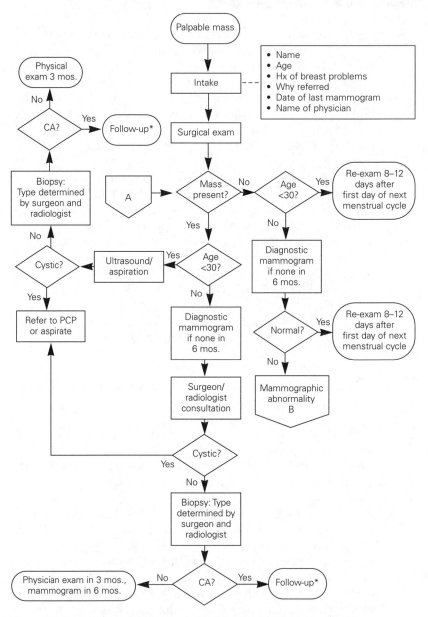

Time of Process: One week from intake to definitive diagnosis

*Follow-up includes setting up an appointment, notification of the primary care physician, and standardization of pathology follow-up (included in educational package). Follow-up is designated by the primary care physician on the referral form.

Published with permission of Advocate Health and Hospital Corporation, Oak Brook, IL.

- The nurse clinical coordinator should facilitate the patient's care by obtaining all necessary clinical and insurance information prior to the patient's visit, providing a seamless approach to the process and decreasing the time to definitive diagnosis.

The steering committee provided a structure for development and implementation of the plan by naming an implementation team and teams responsible for marketing, space, operations, clinical guidelines, and patient education. A chair and facilitator were chosen for those teams, and members of the teams were proposed.

Development Phase   The development phase was initiated by providing an objective or charge to each of the teams designated by the steering committee:

- The implementation team consisted of five key physician stakeholders and a facilitator. This team reworked the vision statement (thus making it their own), wrote the job description for the clinical coordinator (figure 2-6) and the medical director, and developed "seed" algorithms for mammographic abnormality, palpable mass, self-referral, and nipple problem.
- The marketing team was charged with providing an analysis of the current market (SWOT analysis), development of a plan to provide the targeted market with information, creation of tools (including brochures, ad copy, and direct mail), and monitoring the results of marketing.
- The space (physical plant) team was responsible for obtaining a location specifically designated for the center, provision of a space and construction/remodeling plan, and compliance with appropriate regulatory guidelines.
- The operations team was charged with design of registration, insurance verification, intake, follow-up, scheduling, billing, information systems, and budget.
- The clinical guidelines team was assigned the development of algorithms for palpable mass, mammographic abnormality, and self-referral after review of the literature, primary care algorithms in use, and current practice.
- The patient education team was charged with providing a current inventory of information available to patients, designing an education plan for patients, and updating the program with new information as it became available.

The implementation team was the first to be convened. After development of the vision, job descriptions, and seed algorithms, the space, algorithm, and operations teams were convened. The implementation

FIGURE 2-6.   Clinical Coordinator Job Description

Purpose: The Clinical Coordinator of the LGH Breast Center, in cooperation with the Breast Center Medical Director and a multidisciplinary team of health care providers, will facilitate a timely, integrated and coordinated approach to the care of patients with breast disease. It shall be the responsibility of the Clinical Coordinator to triage inquiries, monitor the progress of each individual through the system, by coordinating tests and procedures with alternate sites of care and/or various departments within LGH, acting as a resource for information related to insurance, patient education and options for future care, including the Second Opinion Program. The Clinical Coordinator of the Breast Center will be responsible for overseeing the day-to-day operations of the Center, creating and overseeing utilization of the Breast Center's operational budget and supervising support staff. The Clinical Coordinator will act as a liaison between the Breast Center and other ancillary areas (Surgery, Genetics, Psychology, support groups) to insure that the needs and concerns of the Breast Center patient are addressed.

Accountabilities and Job Activities:

Facilitates a timely, integrated and coordinated approach to patient care:

- Triages all calls to the center, evaluates and prioritizes requests to expedite the provision of quality patient care.
- Works with other sites of care to acquire all necessary information pertinent to provision of care at the Breast Center which may include but not be limited to: obtaining films, test/procedure results, etc.
- Acts as resource for verification of insurance to identify any special requirements necessary to provide timely quality care, i.e., options post Breast Center experience which include but are not limited to: clarification for follow-up treatment, psychological counseling, patient education opportunities provided through the Women's Health Resource Center, and support group activities.
- Acts as resource to facilitate and encourage community outreach.

Oversees operational activities:

- Together with the Manager of Mammography insures appropriate utilization of the Breast Center by supervising patient flow from registration through the procedural areas and identifying opportunities for improvement in process.
- Creates and facilitates utilization of the Breast Center operational budget.
- Hires, supervises and evaluates Breast Center support staff.
- Acts as contact for Advocate Lutheran General Health Partners and other sources of insurance information to keep abreast of the most current policies and benefit requirements.
- Assures that appropriate coding is used for billing purposes.

FIGURE 2-6. (Continued)

- Together with the Medical Director develops policies and procedures according to JCAHO, IDPH, and other regulatory agency guidelines.

Facilitates provision of quality patient care at the LGH Breast Center:

- Remains clinically informed about current diagnostic and treatment methodology by attending and participating in appropriate conferences and seminars.
- Together with the Medical Director, identifies quality indicators and gathers data to measure quality of care utilizing CQI tools.
- Obtains adherence to or deviation from accepted clinical protocols, guidelines, and pathways.
- Participates in teams or committees organized to address issues related to quality of patient care.
- Monitors physician utilization of the Breast Center and presents Medical Director with opportunities for improvement and/or resolution of conflict.

Knowledge, Skills and Abilities

Skills:

- Ability to work well within a multidisciplinary team
- Self-starter
- Advanced knowledge of current diagnostic and treatment methodologies for breast disease
- Prior experience working with protocol/pathway driven environments
- Excellent problem-solving, organizational and communication skills
- Understanding of operational activities (budget prep, etc.)
- Knowledge of computer operations
- Two years experience working with treatment of breast disease
- Two to three years supervisory or leadership experience

Knowledge:

- Bachelors degree or equivalent experience
- Graduate of an accredited school of nursing
- Current Illinois license as a Registered Professional Nurse
- CPR certification

Published with permission of Advocate Health and Hospital Corporation, Oak Brook, IL.

team uncovered a number of questions that were referred to the steering committee for resolution, including:

- Should screening mammograms be done at the center? The recommendation of the implementation team that was approved by the steering committee was to have screening mammograms done at other sites. This decision confirmed that the center would be a referral center for women with breast problems. The inclusion of screening mammography in the center would have greatly increased the volume of patients seen and the space required.
- Would the center accept self-referrals? The implementation and steering committees recommended that self-referrals be accepted. This decision required the development of a process to designate a primary care physician and verify that physician with health maintenance organization and preferred provider organization provider lists.
- How would the hospital interface with the cancer center be managed? Since the center was a unique service line at Lutheran General, the director of the center would be included in the cancer center operations team, and oncology physicians would be included in the development of clinical practice guidelines. The vision of the breast center was clarified to be a diagnostic center.
- Would primary care physicians feel comfortable referring to the center instead of choosing their own preferred surgeon? The consensus was that primary care physicians as a group would be encouraged to refer to the center because of the ease and convenience it provided their patients.

The following issues were resolved by the implementation committee in their initial design:

- Surgeon and radiologist roles were defined by creating an algorithm that provided for a surgeon evaluation for every patient referred to the center and a radiologist consultation for the determination of the type of biopsy.
- The algorithms developed were to be proposed to managed care medical directors as the standard of care for Lutheran General Hospital to reduce the number of contacts, required referrals, and precertifications.
- The chair of the implementation committee was the president-elect of the hospital medical staff and a very respected surgeon who had performed a large volume of breast biopsies. This respected physician met with the division of general surgery to gain agreement that all general surgeons on the medical staff

would participate in providing coverage for the breast center during hours of operation.

- The role of the medical director of the center was determined to be a half-time position with that time designated for provision of clinical leadership in the development of practice guidelines, peer review, administrative leadership in conflict resolution related to physician practice, and responsibility for quality assurance programs.
- The role of the nurse clinical coordinator was determined to be a full-time position requiring an RN with a bachelor's degree who would be responsible for facilitating a coordinated, individualized, and timely approach to patient care, including tracking all patients through the system. (See figure 2-6.)

Implementation Phase   The implementation phase was initiated by beginning the search for candidates for medical director and clinical coordinator. The team felt the final design of the center should have the input of the persons who would carry out its mission.

The space team was convened and began addressing issues related to moving existing personnel, regulatory requirements, and location of equipment. Decisions related to space created a number of delays. The algorithm team was convened and developed consensus algorithms for palpable mass, mammographic abnormality, nipple problem, and self-referral in a single three-hour meeting.

Using the mammography abnormality algorithm as a template, the operations team developed a parallel algorithm of the administrative process (figure 2-7) and a list of issues that included:

- Clarification of the triage process at screening sites and development of a triage form
- Review of the hospital's 1-800 number, including an additional category for the breast center, and triage of problems needing immediate attention
- Verification of insurance for ultrasound instead of using a second referral process (thus eliminating a wait and enabling the patient to have a diagnostic mammogram and ultrasound in the same day)
- Determination of computer hardware and software availability that would interface hospital and physician office systems
- Development of a screening triage form for the center and a process for assignment of a primary care physician for self-referrals
- Determination of location of registration (Breast center patients would register in the waiting area of the center, not the central registration area.)

**FIGURE 2-7.   Algorithm of the Administrative Process
for Mammographic Abnormality**

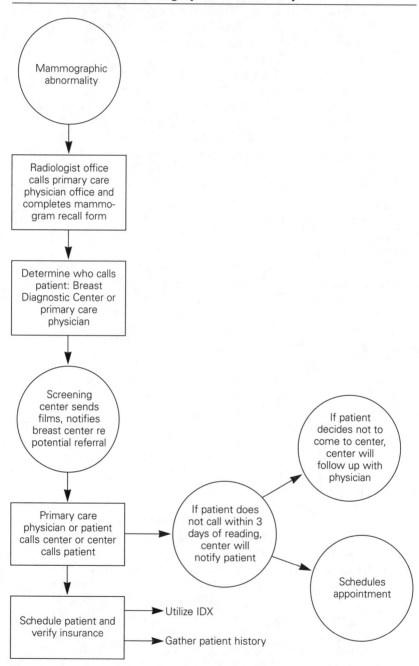

Published with permission of Advocate Health and Hospital Corporation, Oak Brook, IL.

All administrative systems addressed were designed in light of the recommendations contained in the original telephone survey.

The center opened in the summer of 1998, 12 months from the initiation of the project. The medical director and clinical coordinator are responsible for ongoing improvements and refinements. The center will need to track revenue that is generated by it but reported in other departments, such as mammograms, surgical exams, core biopsies, and surgical procedures. Increases in revenue and volume for these procedures can be used in the future to justify the center's continued existence.

Lessons Learned

Following are the key lessons learned from the efforts to develop the breast cancer center.

- Development of clinical practice guidelines does not guarantee their subsequent use. Design of processes and systems of care that support them is required.
- Prior to designing new systems, the systems' quality characteristics should be determined by key customers.
- Clinical guidelines provide a map for clinical care and can be used as a template for development of administrative processes.
- Facilitation of patient care in the present health care environment cannot be assumed without the personal intervention of professional staff assigned to that function.
- A vision developed by senior leadership will need to be reworked by the project team members if they are not included in its initial design.
- The greatest challenges to innovative design of new programs continue to be reimbursement and political concerns.

Contribution of the Nursing Role

The nursing role in the creation of the center changed during the initiative based on the requirements of each phase. For example:

- During the sponsorship phase, the hospital's chief nursing officer acted as an administrative champion, providing personal and organizational support by including the center in the hospital's strategic plan.
- During the development phase, nurses provided facilitation and acted as team members on the six teams that designed the center.

Their input was integral in developing the clinical coordinator's job description, design of space, and clarification of patient education programs.

- During the implementation phase, nursing leadership was again required to support funding and designation of space. The nursing perspective was incorporated into administrative systems that supported the delivery of clinical care.

In all phases, the nursing role required articulate nurses who could form partnerships with physicians, radiology staff, and administration so the nursing perspective could be incorporated into the center's complex clinical and operational processes.

Conclusion

It has been said that the health care system in the United States is poorly named: It is not about health, it is not a system, and it does not care. A "disease management industry" has been suggested as a better description. The breast center project was launched because women seen at Lutheran General Hospital were asking for a system that cared about their health. They were giving voice to the societal need for caregiving.

Diagnosis of breast problems is a highly complex process that is a paradigm for multidisciplinary care. The process raises advocacy issues for women, including the need for information, patient-physician communication, choice of diagnostic approach, psychosocial issues, and insurance problems. An advocate is a helper, counselor, or supporter who defends the best interests of the patient. Advocacy includes ensuring that the patient has access to appropriate care and that she receives high-quality care. The nurse in the role of clinical coordinator of the center was entrusted with the role of advocacy.

The algorithm of the administrative process was designed to be used by the nurse coordinator only as a guide. The coordinator serves as the patient's advocate, designing care to the individual pace and needs of the patient.

Historically, the nursing perspective has integrated issues of holistic caregiving with the maintenance of health. This perspective is most effectively voiced when nurses participate in partnership with administrators and physicians. Effective partnerships are formed when all members share a common vision and a deep appreciation of the knowledge and perspective brought by each partner. The formation of effective partnerships is a challenge, but it is essential for the creation of systems for caregiving.

The role of clinical coordinator for the breast center was essential to its mission because the coordination of care could not be "designed in" to the center without it. A nurse was chosen for that role because the unique perspective of nursing was best suited for the tasks of patient advocacy and the coordination of care. Even if Lutheran General were able to design a seamless process within its walls, the fragmented state of health care outside the walls of the hospital would prevent the center from providing coordination. The nurse who serves as the clinical coordinator provides a place for the patient to share concerns; provides a voice for that patient to the many caregivers, payers, and administrative staff who are involved in her care; and ensures that she has an advocate throughout the entire diagnostic process.

Selected Readings

Breast Center's Redesign Improves Outcomes, Cuts Costs, Attracts MCOs, *Cost Reengineering Report* (July 1997): 103–6.

Durant, John R. How to Organize a Multidisciplinary Clinic for the Management of Breast Cancer, *Surgical Clinics of North America* 70, no. 4 (August 1990): 977–83.

Ganz, Patricia A. Advocating for the Woman with Breast Cancer, *CA-A Cancer Journal for Clinicians* 45 (1995): 114–26.

ICSI Health Care Guideline: Breast Center, Institute for Clinical Systems Integration, Park Nicollet, Minneapolis, MN (1993).

Kneece, Judy, and Cindy Dreher. A Comprehensive Center for the Diagnosis and Treatment of Breast Cancer, *Administrative Radiology* (February 1995): 32–39.

Kornecki, Lynne. Comprehensive Breast Health Centers Offer Convenience for a Multidisciplinary Approach to Treatment, *Chicago Healthcare* (January 1993): 5–7, 28.

Lee, Claudia Z., Cathy Coleman, and John Link. Developing Comprehensive Breast Center, Part One: Introduction and Overview, *The Journal of Oncology Management* 1, no. 1 (May/June 1992): 1–12.

Southwick, Karen. In Super-Competitive Minneapolis Region, Park Nicollet's Cross-Functional Clinical Teams Streamline Outpatient Care Services, *Strategies for Healthcare Excellence* 6, no. 7 (July 1993): 1–6.

3

Developing a Winning Business Plan

Mae Taylor Moss, MS, MSN, RN, FAAN

M ark Twain wrote "Clothes make the man," and then added, "Naked people have little or no influence in society." We know it is true, yet many nurse entrepreneurs and executives go naked into the world of work without the "clothing" of an excellent business plan. The business plan, like the clothes an executive wears, portrays the style of performance, depicts the attention to detail the executive will give to the initiative proposed, and provides an indication of the writer's organizational powers and critical thinking skills. Like clothes, the business plan makes the first impression. It apprises investors about the potential marketability of the services, and, in the end, it serves as a guide to the business operator for what has to be done in what order. Within an organization, a business plan can ensure that partners, employees, and even subcontractors understand the company's direction, and it can become a mechanism for consensus building in a management team.[1]

The writing in a business plan can make or break the plan's acceptance. Once it is in the hands of venture capitalists, bank officers, or, for an internal business plan, superiors within an organization, the report is the only representative the idea has. If the idea is not expressed well, readers are likely to think it is a bad idea. A writer cannot stand beside each reader, ready to answer questions. The report must stand on its own.

This chapter reviews the basic sections of a business plan and explains their purpose. It also includes a guide to business plan software and manufacturers' Web sites for those comfortable with composing on the keyboard and wary of preparing a business plan from scratch. A case study of a business plan developed by the University of Iowa Hospitals and Clinics Department of Nursing and Patient Care Services is presented at the end of the chapter.

THE BUSINESS PLAN

Every business plan is unique, so every writer must shape the basic elements to meet specific needs. The business plan includes:

- Executive summary
- Introduction
- Business profile
- Marketing plan
- Operational plan
- Organizational plan
- Financial plan
- Conclusion
- Appendices

Executive Summary and Introduction

The executive summary condenses to one page the critical elements of the entire business plan. Some writers allow the summary to stretch to as many as five pages, perhaps because they fear it will be the only part of the report that will be read carefully.[2] Inasmuch as it is a summary of the whole, it should be written when the document is complete. It should not describe what is found in each section of the plan; it should restate it. Because some investors request only the executive summary for a preliminary evaluation, its importance is magnified.

The introduction's purpose is to set the stage for the production about to unfold. That means clearly identifying such major elements as the business and principals by name, describing the business or service or product provided, and placing those things and people within geographic and market boundaries. Each element should be identified by its full formal name. If the business name is long, the writer can parenthetically identify a short name for it, including calling it, as many lawyers do, *the company* or *the partnership*, and consistently referring to it by that name throughout the proposal.

This section is also the place to define what problems the proposal will solve and to delineate the scope of the plan. A brief history that explains the relationship of the principals, the background of demand, an interpretation of the economic situation, or other background information that clarifies the present is a critical part of explaining the solution offered by the business plan. Knowing the scope helps readers know what to expect: Will the proposal make projections for two years or five or ten? Will it discuss citywide or statewide or global services? Will it be a short-range or long-range plan? Like the most helpful of personal introductions, which include a friendly statement characterizing or identifying the person being introduced, the business plan introduction may highlight specific features—a balance sheet, forecast of earnings, timeline, or organizational chart—that the writer thinks may be of special interest to the reader. Letting the reader know that the forecast of earnings indicates recovery of investment in less than, say, four years, that the timeline shows getting into foreign markets is feasible within a fiscal year, or that impressive letters of support are in the appendix may help jump-start the reader's positive perception of the proposal. Like the executive summary, the introduction should be drafted after the rest of the plan has been written.

Business Profile

In the business profile, the business plan writer gives an overview of the business that includes, but is not limited to, the following:

- A definition of the company and a one-sentence statement of its purpose, services, and products (a mission statement)
- A description of what the business wants to be—its ideal for the future (a vision statement)
- Brief descriptions of the major projects, services, or products

The definition should be simple enough that whoever reads the plan can repeat it. This definition may be the mission statement, which answers the question of what the business is, who it serves, what the purposes are for which it exists, and what makes it unique or significant. What follows next is the vision statement—a description of what the business wants to be. Then the writer's job is describing how the business intends to get from what it is to what it wants to be. That, in essence, is the business plan.

Some of the topics introduced briefly in this section are those that the plan describes in more detail later. These include:

- The market and environment assessments
- Facilities
- Personnel (including management)
- Scheduling
- Cost requirements
- History of the project

Discussing the background or history along with the description of the business is natural because these elements follow logically, and this puts the history in mind as the description of the business is presented.

The description of the business tells how it will be operated to achieve a stated aim. This aim may be achieving sales of a certain number of units, serving a stated number of patients per unit time, or meeting a specific need. The description of actions the business will take may be spelled out in terms of phases or of typical practice or may be a broad overview of services performed. The plan may also be divided into short- and long-range plans, especially if the activities of the operation may change over time or the percentage of time devoted to specific activities is expected to shift over time.

One company's business plan, for example, used one table to explain the analytical components of some of the consulting services the company provided, indicating the products the hospital would gain from the analysis, and another table to show the benefits that would accrue to the institution once new processes were in place. Also, to generally explain the company's consulting approach, it used a diagram to illustrate each action graphically as one step that led to the next. In the text, it was explained what tasks had to be completed to move from one step to another and what the relationships were between the steps.

The writer may preview the remaining sections of the plan and present a concise and cohesive expression of the business's aims and abilities to achieve them by providing a brief explanation of the following:

- The appropriateness and special features of the business's facilities
- The key personnel critical in achieving the goals set out
- The continuum of achievement marked with significant milestones (a timeline)
- The cost

If any outstanding intellectual property is held (patents, licenses, or trademarks), it should be mentioned in this section.

Marketing Plan

Many consider the marketing plan the make-or-break proposal component and absolutely critical to the success of the plan. In it, the writer must define the market, assess the market and environment, analyze the competition, and create and delineate the marketing strategy.

Defining the Market and the Opportunity   Although many entrepreneurs focus on their products or services and can demonstrate exceptional expertise, their efforts are useless unless they can show credibly that demand exists and that they understand the market. Demonstrating a need for the product or services requires identifying a market and characterizing the possibilities of mining it. The discussion should define the scope of the market, both in a broad sense and a more narrow sense in which the writer identifies and delineates primary and secondary markets.

Marketing has been defined as the practice of the three Rs: research, reach, and retain.[3] In this discussion, the emphasis remains on research: understanding the environment in which the product or services will be offered and how the proposed products or services compare to those of competitors. According to one accounting firm, venture capitalists look to the marketing plan as a very significant indicator of the likelihood of the enterprise's success.[4]

Assessing the Market and the Environment   The assessment of the current market and environment provides an opportunity for the authors of business plans to show that they are acutely aware of their product's market and the environment in which they are operating. The plan should include both geographic and other demographic indicators:

- Assessment of the current geographic market, including identifying both primary and secondary markets (for example, by zip code)
- Assessment of the market within a city (or metropolitan statistical areas), a state, a U.S. region, the United States, and around the globe (if applicable)
- Assessment of the customer by demographics

A visiting nurse service provider, for example, would want to know which geographic areas provided most of its patients (51–80 percent, for example), which areas were secondary (20–49 percent), and how its market penetration fared comparatively with other similar service providers. It might also want to identify patients by age, sex, type of payer, diagnosis, and origin of referral.

In the analysis of the service, industry, or product environment, it is important to identify the pressures affecting the business at hand most dramatically. For example, a provider of alternative medicine would want to cite those trends indicating acceptance of fees by third-party payers and any research indicating favorable leanings toward alternative health providers. A group of urological oncologists, for example, would want to produce predictions of new cancer cases relative to their specialty for their metropolitan area and estimate how many of those cases would be treated by their group (estimated market share).

Specific government regulations and the broader political and social climate should also be explored to characterize their influence on the service or product environment. The effect of government regulations or rules governing Medicare and Medicaid can be profound on marketability. For example, increases in the number of women 65 years old and older undergoing mammography were dramatic after the government approved funding of the screening. Political and social trends also affect personal decision making. Broader powers bestowed by the national and state governments on advanced nurse practitioners have implications for providers seeking the most cost-effective means of providing certain health care services formerly supplied only by physicians. Today, because of patients' interest in participating more fully in their health care, pharmaceutical companies create advertising appeals for prescription medicines for general interest magazines as well as medical journals. How other determinants, such as convenience, technological innovation, and reputation affect marketability should also be explored if market research is available.

Gauging customer satisfaction remains an important way to determine how the product or service meets customer requirements and to interpret changes in the company's fortunes. Some hospitals have external companies perform their customer satisfaction surveys and then, with positive results, broadcast their success. Performing these assessments themselves might subject the findings to claims of bias.

Analyzing the Competition   In almost all endeavors, competition exists. Ask the elementary school child in a foot race, the high school girl in love with the football quarterback, or any assistant vice president at a large bank. They all feel the competition. In the business plan, the writer must identify the competition and then explain how, against those competitors, advantages can be maximized and disadvantages minimized.

To provide a fair look at the competition, answer for the reader how each competitor is similar to and how each is different from the business proposed. Begin by answering the following questions:

- How many businesses provide the same or similar goods or services?
- How are they similar and how are they different from the business in the business plan?
- Where do competitors rank in the industry?
- What are the major players' competitive positions in terms of market share or other factors?
- How does their position compare to that of the business of the business plan?

One simple way to compare your company to others in the market is to construct a table. (For an example, see table 3-1.) Information in the table should not be duplicated in the text. The text should highlight

TABLE 3-1. Comparison of Competitors

Company	Size (staff)	Age (years)	Expertise	Scope	Strengths	Weaknesses
ABC, Inc. New York, NY	250	15	Hospital	National	• Largest in industry • Diverse expertise • Four nationwide offices • Physician consultants	• High fees • Limited depth • High staff turnover
John Doe, Inc. Chicago, IL	35	25	OR	International	• Extensive database • Benchmarking services • Excellent reputation	• Low fees • Poor management • High staff turnover
Acme Health Care Dallas, TX	20	12	OR	National	• Large nursing staff • Limited focus	• Staff difficult to recruit and retain • Nondiversified
XYZ Management New York, NY	90	4	Automation	International	• Strong central office • Strong technology group	• Limited OR expertise • Staff broad without depth • Conservatism stifling growth
My Company, Inc. San Francisco, CA	2	<1	OR	International	• Strong OR focus • Broad experience • Service depth • Physician consultants	• New company • Little name recognition • Fledgling fee structure

facts presented in the table, guiding the reader to what is significant. The reader will want to know who was included and why they were selected. Well-known competitors who are omitted must have their absence explained. Similar factors on which to compare companies include products, product benefits, advertising and promotion efforts, sales, and distribution.[5] Those in direct competition (offering the same service or product to the same target market) and those in indirect competition (offering the same service or product to a different target market) can be included. The entrepreneur can use this section to distinguish his or her business from its competitors. The aim here should be to show product or service strengths, indicating enough breadth without seeming shallow. Experts recommend explaining benefits of products or services substantively without being overly technical.[6] Being concise scores extra points.

The focus here should be on distinctive competencies that set the proposed business apart. These could be in terms of competitive position, noteworthy capabilities, or existing relationships that translate into meaningful support and customer convenience. For example, establishment of a free-standing advanced practice nursing clinic in orthopedics might benefit from setting up business in a building where other tenants were in related or supporting practices—physical therapists, a magnetic resonance imaging center, and a rehabilitation center with whirlpool facilities and exercise machines, for example.

Creating a Marketing Strategy   Mapping a marketing plan requires the same attention to detail as creating a care map. Both require a keen understanding of the consumer (in the case of the care map, the patient), and both require being able not only to forecast the most likely outcomes but also to think ahead and decide what responses will be made to atypical cases. In essence, the marketing strategy, which is based on the following three issues, is an explanation of how the proposed product or services will meet a need.

- *Identifying and characterizing the need.* To identify and characterize what niche of a market the proposed product or services will fill, the writer must pair the market and opportunity definition presented previously with research, effectively demonstrating how the elements are, like gears, synchronized and working together to propel the proposed endeavor forward. Research, whether formal or anecdotal, supports assertions of need, provides a basis for pricing and financial forecasts, and helps target communication. Businesses can pinpoint regional populations by income, average cost of home, age, even length of average commute, and many other variables. Once research is under way, keeping abreast of findings may spare the business wasted effort and lost revenue.

- *Predicting the scope of the need.* Calculating the breadth and depth of the need involves developing a pricing and distribution strategy. Some business plans place sections describing pricing, delivery or distribution, and communication before research, but discussing research first allows the writer to substantiate choices in these other areas with findings from research. Research can identify how the proposed product or services will compare in price to those of competitors and unique ways to package the goods for different customers (for example, insured patients and managed care companies). Pricing schedules, if complex, may require documentation in the appendix. Demographic profiles and government and marketing statistical reports can foster ideas about delivery and distribution. Is access to the product or services convenient? Is it in line with customer expectations? Remember that potential financial backers may contact proposed distributors to determine their view of the potential success of the product.[7] Research also fuels sales forecasts. Though financial reports fall later in the business plan scheme, projecting growth at this point may be important to demonstrate the appropriateness of the level of planning, an awareness of industry trends, and a sensitivity to market-entry timing.
- *Communicating how the product or services meet the need.* Advertising and public relations are two formal ways businesses use to communicate with customers. Communicating with the purchaser to generate sales may be as direct as telephone solicitation or as indirect as engendering good will by participation in civic or charity efforts, such as a walk or run for a national not-for-profit agency like the American Heart Association. Direct marketing can be expensive, while public relations efforts or publicity—advising media of events or developments at an institution—can be inexpensive or cost nothing. The size of the advertising budget may dictate the size of this section, but in addition to describing methods, naming media, and justifying why they were chosen, business plan writers may want to suggest how these efforts might be augmented in the future.

Operational Plan

In the section describing the operational plan, the writer defines the parts of the operation and how they will work together. In technical texts, drawings that show all the parts of a machine separated but positioned relative to their neighboring parts are called *exploded drawings*. With these drawings, it is easy to see each individual part yet understand its relation to other parts. Business plans, like these drawings, can delineate each major part of the operation producing the product or services as well as show how the parts operate together.

What the operational plan demonstrates is that the writer has bridged the gap from idea or design to pragmatic implementation. That doesn't mean that every technical detail has to be explained. Relegate complex presentations to the appendix. The careful writer proceeds with caution, avoiding extreme scientific jargon yet explaining the idea in clear terms.

If a company is proposing a specialty clinic, for example, the business plan would describe the services the clinic will offer and include the critical care pathways and clinical practice guidelines that describe the protocols to be followed. A diagram of the patient-flow process would also identify the relationships between processes and the points of interface. A part of understanding the patient flow is understanding how the following components will function: appointment scheduling, registration, medical history taking and examination, diagnostic testing, treatment, patient education, and follow-up appointments or calls. Demonstrating a clear plan for what happens next—how the business services component will process charges, collect fees, and follow up on delinquent accounts—tells the reader that these aspects have been carefully thought out.

The physical plant—the facilities available for carrying out the services—must be described so that it is clear that the square footage, equipment, and location are sufficient to meet the demands of providing the services. A floor plan and a map of traffic flow can show how the space will accommodate staff and patients.

Organizational Plan

The human resources plan must show that the business has carefully assessed the company's requirements, objectively evaluated the principals' strengths and weaknesses, and created a staffing plan that balances requirements with personnel. Two essential elements of the organizational plan are the principals, or founders, of the enterprise and the organization of management and staff, usually presented as a chart.

Key personnel usually include the founders and the top staff they have hired to operate the business. Under the staff will be administrative personnel and support staff. Business plan writers will want to make clear when (and perhaps at what salary) these staff members come on board. Projections may be for three to five years. For clinical organizations, staffing ratios should be reported. Brief biographical descriptions may be included in the text and complete employment résumés in the appendix. What is important here is demonstrating the competence of the group assembled and the match of their skills or experience to the job at hand. For the future, the plan may want to project what skills mix may be required, what positions could be combined (if any), and what new employees might be required by new technology. The organizational chart will show the relationships of the major players to one another and the relationship of any governing board of directors or advisory board to the operation.

Financial Plan

The financial plan has been called the heart of the business plan, probably because the enterprise may live or die by its strength.[8] It is the broad view of how the company expects to fare financially. Unless the business plan is for an existing business anticipating expansion or acquisition, the figures will be projections and therefore require a statement of assumptions on which the projections are based. These assumptions take on critical importance because, if they are not reliable, the projections will not be.

The documents required for this section include:

- A profit and loss statement, which calculates projected income against the cost of operations to show the gain or loss of the business. Table 3-2 is a simple example that does not include tax considerations.
- A projected cash flow statement, which indicates the business's net financial position based on income and disbursements (table 3-3).
- A balance sheet, which reports the financial standing of a business on a specific date. It indicates the assets (what the company owns), the liabilities (what the company owes), and the capital (value of ownership) (table 3-4).

Financial projections are by month for the first two to three years and then annually for up to five or ten years.

Cash flow statements begin with a beginning cash balance (cash on hand). To that is added collections: sales, collections from credit accounts, loans received, and any interest earned. Only sales is included in a projected income statement. Subtracted are the disbursements: gross wages and payroll expenses, supplies, repair and maintenance costs, transportation expenses, advertising and marketing expenditures, and other expenses such as rent and utilities. Depreciation is also included. The disbursements are subtracted from the collections, resulting in a cash balance or deficiency.

TABLE 3-2. Specialty Consulting Profit and Loss Statement (in Thousands)

	Jan.	Feb.	Mar.	Apr.	May	Jun.	Jul.	Aug.	Sep.	Oct.	Nov.	Dec.
Revenue (sales)												
Hospital A	$ 35	$ 35	$ 35		$ 10	$10	$35	$50	$40			
Hospital B	90	90	90		45	45	15	15				
Hospital C					25	25	25	10				
Hospital D				$90						$ 30	$ 30	$ 30
Total revenue	125	125	125	90	80	80	75	75	40	30	30	30
Cost of sales												
Salary/benefits	100	100	100	66	66	66	35	35	35	35	35	35
Supplies		1			1			1		1		
Travel	16	16	16	16	12	12	12	17				2
Office	2	2	2	2	2	2	2	2	2	2	2	2
Total cost of sales	118	119	118	84	81	80	49	55	37	38	37	39
Profit (or loss)	$ 7	$ 6	$ 7	$ 6	$(−1)	$ 0	$26	$20	$ 3	$(−8)	$(−7)	$(−9)

The balance sheet is the "snapshot" of the business at a specific time, and it shows the business's weaknesses and strengths at that particular time (table 3-4). It is a summary of the financial transactions of the operation.

These three documents make up the core of the financial section. Some planners add an index to indebtedness—the debt-to-assets ratio—which is total liabilities divided by total assets. For example, if a company has total liabilities of $25,000 but has assets of $50,000, it has a 1:2 debt-to-assets ratio. Another index—the debt-to-equity ratio—describes what is owed in relation to the owners' equity in the company (total liabilities divided by total equity). A sole proprietor would have 100 percent equity; therefore, if the liabilities were $25,000 and the equity was $100,000, the debt-to-equity ratio for that owner would be 1:4. Remember that these reports will not only help sell a prospective business but, with proper updating, help manage it once it is on track.

TABLE 3-3. Specialty Consulting Cash Flow Statement

	Month 1
Starting cash	$1,125
Cash in (receipts)	
Cash sales (collections)	500
Paid receivables	500
Other	0
Total cash in	1,000
Cash out (disbursements)	
Rent	350
Wages/benefits	500
Other	0
Total cash out	850
Ending balance	1,275
Change (cash flow)	150

TABLE 3-4. Specialty Consulting Balance Sheet

Specialty Consulting Balance Sheet
31 December 199–

Assets		Liabilities and Capital	
Cash	$34,000	Accounts payable	$ 6,400
Accounts receivable	5,000	Notes payable	60,700
Property	78,400	Total liabilities	71,100
Total assets	$117,400	Principals' capital	46,400
		Total liabilities and capital	$117,400

Plan Conclusion and Appendices

"The difference between a winning and losing proposal," one textbook writer said, "is often an intangible: confidence."[9] That confidence is built into each section intrinsically, so that by the end, the conclusion that the plan deserves support should be self-evident. That leaves the writer the task of simply summarizing the venture's virtues at the end.

Supporting documentation that is too technical, too lengthy, or inappropriate for inclusion in the text should find a home in the back matter of the report. Résumés, the owner's personal financial statement, letters of reference, contracts, equipment documentation, legal agreements, marketing brochures, and maps in the appendix can support claims and arguments made within the plan without disturbing its flow.

BUSINESS PLAN SOFTWARE

For those who are wary of preparing their own business plans, a selection of software exists that can help create a business plan based on templates and canned language (table 3-5). *Home Office Computing* prepared a comparison of nine packages to help writers launch their businesses, but other reviews also offer guidance.[10] Known as part of the software market niche called *MBA-ware* or *smart business software*, these packages guide the writer though every part of plan preparation.[11] In addition, some of the manufacturers' Web sites offer expertise and advice once the product is purchased. Presented in table 3-5 is a rough guide to some recent plans; before buying, check the manufacturers' Web sites for new editions or upgrades and more reviews. Palo Alto Software offers at its Web site (http://www.bplans.com) sample business plans as examples.

EXTERNAL AND INTERNAL BUSINESS PLANS

The focus of this description has been business plans intended for external review, but big medical centers rely on the same kind of presentations to create new clinics, services, or other endeavors within their own walls. Perhaps foremost, it is important to demonstrate that the mission and vision of the proposed entity are in line with those of the larger institution. That means, too, that the goals and objectives of the proposed project should be consistent with those of the institution and that the means of achieving them are in line with its policies and practices. Overall, the plan should reflect a sensitivity of the part to the whole: the physical location on the larger campus, conformity with budgetary calendar and personnel grades and salaries, and a plan for involving or advising significant institutional personnel with responsibilities relative to the project.

TABLE 3-5. Business Plan Software Packages

Software Package	Review
BizPlan Builder ($99) by Jian www.jianusa.com 800.346.5426 (Mac version also available)	• "... leading business planning program"[12] • A help to "both novices and seasoned pros"[13] • A variety of templates with financial plan spreadsheets[14]
Plan Write ($130) and Plan Write Expert Edition ($229) by Business Resource Software www.brsinc.com 800.423.1228	• Template plus analysis and marketing strategies; goes to "real life concerns of running a business"[15] • Rated #1 of nine packages—a Best Buy[16]
Smart Business Plan ($89) by American Institute for Financial Research www.smartonline.com 800.578.900	• Easy to use interface; can combine product and services approaches[17]
Business Plan Pro ($99) Palo Alto Software www.palo-alto.com 800.229.7526	• "Flexible interface, a variety of templates"[18] • "... really shines ... in the quality of the finished business plan"[19]
Business Plan Toolkit for Macintosh ($80–$150) Palo Alto Software www.palo-alto.com 800.229.7526	• "... documentation is especially helpful"; integrates with Word and Excel best but also works with ClarisWorks and Microsoft Works[20]

Note: Reviews were for various versions. Consult the manufacturers' Web sites for the most up-to-date versions.

CONCLUSION

The well-written business plan, like a well-chosen and perfectly pressed suit, presents an executive impression of competence. Inclusion of the standard elements, in a thorough and thoughtful presentation, demonstrates knowledge about the endeavor proposed, a keen, well-researched view of the market, and willingness to grapple with the details in order to reduce risk.

References

1. A. McKeon. Writing a "Killer" Business Plan, conference presentation, Younger Technologists Forum, Atlanta (1997).

2. J. A. Covello and B. J. Hazelgren. *The Complete Book of Business Plans: Simple Steps to Writing a Powerful Business Plan* (Naperville, IL: Sourcebooks, 1995).

3. L. Pinson and J. Jinnett. *Anatomy of a Business Plan*, 3d ed. (Chicago: Upstart Publishing, 1996).

4. E. S. Siegel, B. R. Ford, and J. M. Bornstein. *The Ernst & Young Business Plan Guide*, 2d ed. (New York: John Wiley, 1993), p. 63.

5. Ibid., p. 79.

6. Ibid., p. 66.

7. Ibid., p. 86.

8. Covello and Hazelgren.

9. S. E. Pauley. *Technical Report Writing* Today, 2d ed. (Boston: Houghton Mifflin, 1979), p. 172.

10. In addition to those sources cited in table 3-5, see also J. S. Dawson. Business-Plan Templates, *MacWorld* 12 (1995): 61.

11. Smarterware, *Fortune* 134 (winter 1997): 104.

12. R. Mendosa. Where's Your Plan? *Hispanic Business* 19 (1997): 46.

13. Smarterware, p. 104.

14. J. T. Patz. Step-by-Step Business Planning, *Home Office Computing* 14 (1996): 120–27.

15. T. K. Muhammad. Plan Write from the Start, *Black Enterprise* 42 (November 1997): 42, 44.

16. Patz, p. 127.

17. M. Hogan. Business Planning, *PC World* 15 (1992): 180–81.

18. Ibid., p. 180.

19. Patz, p. 125.

20. Ibid.

CASE STUDY: WOUND OSTOMY CONTINENCE BUSINESS PLAN

Beverly Folkedahl, RN, CWOCN

The University of Iowa Hospitals and Clinics (UIHC) Department of Nursing and Patient Care Services in Iowa City developed a business plan to outline and support expansion of wound, ostomy, and skin care services to external agencies in the area. The Wound Ostomy and Continence (WOC) Nursing Service is designed to respond to market demand for specialized nursing care for patients with selected disorders of the gastrointestinal, genitourinary, and integumentary systems. It is a component of the organized system of nursing services provided through the UIHC Clinical Enterprise, which is committed to build on its traditional missions of patient care, education, and research; innovation in the delivery of health care; adapting the organization to succeed in a changing environment; and working collaboratively as partners with the people, communities, and organizations it serves.

This case study describes the UIHC business plan for the nursing service, outlining its purpose, marketing strategy, related issues, financial considerations, and the benefits and risks of beginning the new business venture. It also presents lessons learned from the process and discusses future issues.

Plan Alignment with Institutional Mission/Vision

The University of Iowa Hospitals and Clinics serves as the teaching hospital and comprehensive health care center for the state of Iowa, thereby promoting the health of the citizens of Iowa. The UIHC, in concert with the University of Iowa health science colleges, functions in support of health care professionals and organizations in Iowa and other states by:

- Offering a broad spectrum of clinical services to all patients cared for within the center and through its outreach programs
- Serving as the primary teaching hospital for the university
- Providing a base for innovative research to improve health care

The UIHC and the College of Medicine, working as partners to provide high-quality health care, share a clear vision for continuing excellence built around the four key concepts of tradition, innovation, adaptation, and collaboration.

The Department of Nursing and Patient Care Services provides the administrative structure and decision framework through which nursing works with other clinical and hospital departments to manage UIHC's capacity to provide patient and family care and related nursing education, research, and nursing informative services across the UIHC system.

Business Profile

The objective was to build an organized system of WOC nursing services, including prevention, health maintenance, therapeutic intervention, and rehabilitation services to respond to market demand.

Strategic Intent of the Service   The strategic intent of the UIHC WOC nursing service was to provide the following:

- WOC services to agencies and facilities that currently do not have them
- Positive collaborative working relationships between the service and community-based agencies and facilities
- Incremental revenue to the University of Iowa Clinical Enterprise

Market   Iowa's population of citizens over 65 is the third largest in the nation, and Iowa leads the nation in residents 85 and older. The 15.4 percent of Iowa's population age 65 and older accounted for 47 percent of patient days in Iowa hospitals in 1992. This population experiences disorders of the gastrointenstinal, genitourinary, and integumentary systems such as:

- Stomas
- Draining wounds
- Fistulas/tubes
- Vascular ulcers
- Presssure ulcers
- Neuropathic ulcers
- Incontinence

In 1994, long-term care facilities had a national pressure ulcer rate ranging from 2.4 to 23 percent. Elderly patients admitted for femoral fractures had a 66 percent incidence, and critical care patients had an incidence of 33 percent.[1]

Approximately 72 nurses are currently certified to provide wound, ostomy, and continence services in the state of Iowa. However, within Johnson, Muscatine, Cedar, Washington, Louisa, Iowa, and Keokuk counties, WOC services are limited to only three certified WOC nurses actively employed. WOC-certified nurses employed at two community hospitals in Cedar Rapids (Linn County) have a limited number of contracts with long-term care facilities in some of the above-mentioned counties.

In June 1996, a local community hospital and its subsidiary home care agency requested WOC nursing services from the UHIC Department of Nursing and Patient Care Services. The community hospital wanted to replace the services of a WOC nurse who had relocated. After a prolonged and unsuccessful attempt to recruit an external candidate, the hospital administration decided to explore the potential of subcontracting for WOC services. In February 1997, after several meetings to clarify customer need and UIHC capacity to respond, the community hospital and UIHC Department of Nursing and Patient Care Services entered into a contractual agreement to provide WOC hospital and home health consultant services, leaving UIHC free to contract directly with nursing homes that the hospital had previously covered through its home care agency.

Specific Services Offered   The certified WOC nurse possesses the advanced level of knowledge and highly technical skills necessary to provide direct care or consult regarding nursing care of wounds, fistulas, ulcers, stomas, and incontinence amenable to nursing intervention. Following are useful definitions of the conditions requiring WOC nurse care:

- Debridement: Removal of avascular tissue
- Draining wounds: Any type of wound, acute or chronic, requiring protective or containment dressings
- Fistula: An abnormal passage between two organs or structures
- Incontinence: Inability to control urine or stool
- Neuropathic ulcer: A wound resulting from the loss of sensory, motor, or autonomic pathways
- Pressure ulcer: A wound resulting from excessive pressure on tissue causing tissue necrosis
- Stomas: A surgically created opening used to transport urine or stool from the body
- Vascular ulcer: A wound resulting from inadequate or insufficient circulation

Market Plan for the Service

WOC nursing services are used in acute, long-term, outpatient, and home health care settings. Patients who require this highly specialized type of nursing care range in age from pre-term infants to the elderly. Each age group may be found in any setting and each requires a unique skill set to deal with its problems. The WOC nurse is well equipped educationally to provide this patient care.

UIHC WOC nursing services were to be offered to acute-care hospitals, long-term care facilities, primary-care offices, UIHC outreach clinics, and home care agencies in the surrounding area. Local home care agencies and long-term care facilities frequently contacted UIHC WOC nurses to request assistance with specific patient problems. These patients had been seen at UIHC without charge to either the patient or the agency. It was recommended that UIHC investigate a mechanism to charge for this service.

Market Direction   Because WOC nurses at UIHC were initially contacted by an external agency, the market was evident. Two Johnson County long-term care facilities, one Muscatine County facility, and one Van Buren County facility had already requested WOC nursing services for their respective agencies. These contacts were all initiated externally without advertising. Our intent was to send query letters to other potential users of this service.

Key Competitors   Key competitors to the UIHC WOC services are:

- Physicians
   —Primary care
   —Dermatology
   —Plastic surgery
- Physical therapists
- Product company representatives (who provide consulting as a value-added service with product use)
- WOC nurses in Linn, Scott, and Henry counties

Potential competitors also include freestanding wound care clinics operated by national corporations. Such facilities currently operate in Davenport and Des Moines.

Target Markets   The targeted counties are Johnson, Cedar, Iowa, Keokuk, Louisa, Muscatine, and Washington. These counties are in close proximity to and have a relationship with UIHC and lack available WOC nurses. Initial communications were directed to the agencies in Johnson, Washington, and Muscatine counties, all within a 90-mile radius of Iowa City—the program's primary market. After development of contracts with the primary markets, the secondary markets of Cedar, Iowa, Keokuk, and Louisa will be targeted. Other secondary markets include managed care companies, insurance providers, and health maintenance organizations.

Table 3-6 outlines the number of potential markets for WOC nurse services in the target areas.

Products and Services Offered

The WOC nurse provides the following services:

- Direct care for patients with selected disorders of the gastro-intestinal, genitourinary, and integumentary systems
- Consultant services to agencies to assist the primary caregiver
- Educational offerings to agency staff
- Product evaluation
- Policy and protocol development
- Assistance with state regulatory compliance

Contracts for service fees are negotiated with the agency. Because the UIHC WOC nurses are not advanced RN practitioners, direct fee-for-service patient billing is not an option at this time.

Training

A WOC nurse is a baccalaureate-prepared RN who has completed an accredited Wound Ostomy Continence Nurses Society (WOCN) educational program. Seven accredited programs are currently available in the United States. These programs provide in-depth education in the care of the patient with wounds, ostomies, or incontinence. Following successful completion of the program, the WOC nurse has the opportunity to certify in the specialty. This certification is offered by the Wound Ostomy Continence Nursing Certification Board. In order to maintain certification, the WOC nurse must repeat the certification process every five years. All WOC nurses at UIHC are certified.

Timeline of Service Provision

It is anticipated that the primary market of Johnson, Washington, and Muscatine counties will be contracted within six months. Secondary markets in Cedar, Louisa, Iowa, and Keokuk will be developed after that in three-month intervals. By using this gradual roll-out, we are able to judge the time demands on the nurses inherent with travel to outside agencies.

TABLE 3-6. Potential Markets for WOC Nurses

County	Acute	Skilled	Intermediate	Home Care
Cedar	0	2	4	1
Johnson	2	5	8	5
Iowa	1	1	5	2
Keokuk	1	1	5	1
Louisa	0	0	3	1
Muscatine	1	2	5	1
Washington	1	2	2	5
Total	6	13	32	16

Pricing Policies of the Service

Fees are negotiated with each type of agency. The community hospital pays UIHC a mutually agreed upon fixed price for hospital and home care visits. Our contracts with local long-term care agencies provide for an hourly fee calculated on total time, including travel, of each visit.

Organizational Structure of the WOC Service

UIHC's WOC nursing service has a separate cost center within the Department of Nursing and Patient Care Services. It is organized within the Medical-Surgical I Clinical Nursing Division that houses the majority of inpatient populations with need for WOC services. Reorganization of the service from within the Medical-Surgical I Division may need to be considered.

Contractual Services for the WOC Nurse

To meet market demand for WOC services both within UIHC and externally, the Department of Nursing and Patient Care Services subcontracts with the local county health agency to provide a certified WOC nurse on a 60 percent basis. This is mutually beneficial. However, it is anticipated we will need to employ a WOC-certified nurse full time to meet the needs of UIHC patients as the number of external contracts increases.

Operations

In a new service, consideration must be given to daily operational tasks. Record keeping and communication tools are vital to the success of the service and require time, personnel, and financial support.

Record and Communications   The WOC nurses keep accurate records of both internal and external activities. Expanded computer support to develop a systematic record of visits is vital to the success of the program. Each WOC nurse must have computer access to the activity of the service. Because the WOC nurses are currently not geographically located in the same area of the hospital, computer access facilitates communication and provides for continuity.

Service Start-Up Needs   The service requires clerical support to do billing and maintain financial records. Initially, other equipment required by the service included:

- A camera for documentation of wounds
- Blood pressure equipment
- A Doppler to check pulses and calculate ankle brachial index
- Cellular phone

The integrated call system was notified about the service so calls and contacts could be directed to the correct service.

Roles and Responsibilities Three WOC nurses currently work at UIHC, including:

- Advanced practice nurse (APN), 90 percent appointment, WOC nurse since 1983
- APN, who devotes approximately 50 percent of her full-time oncology clinical nurse specialist position to WOC services, WOC nurse since 1993
- Specialty nurse clinician, 60 percent contracted appointment beginning July 1997, WOC nurse since 1992

Total WOC nursing experience is 23 years. Calls are directed to the APN. She triages the calls and the WOC nurse with the most appropriate skill mix is assigned. Each WOC nurse is responsible for documentation according to facility requirements and entering the appropriate information on the UIHC records for documentation and billing purposes.

Each WOC nurse is certified in the specialty and has a professional responsibility to remain current. This is accomplished through involvement with the professional organization on a state and national level and continuing education attendance at appropriate conferences. This activity should be supported by the department.

Risks and Benefits of the Service

Because of perceptions in the private sector regarding academic health science centers as competitors rather than "free" statewide resources, agencies that currently employ WOC nurses may see expansion of this service outside UIHC as a threat. With that in mind, the new service is not marketed in areas already covered by established WOC nurses. WOC nurses in Iowa have historically had an excellent working relationship and this program will not interfere with that.

Other risks and benefits include:

- *Employee-partner relationships:* This service need not conflict with new alliances being formed by UIHC and the Clinical Enterprise. To avoid the possibility, the director of nursing and patient care services reviews all potential agencies prior to the contract proposal.

- *New-product risk:* Agency decision makers are unfamiliar with the function and role of the WOC nurse. Thus, it is imperative that the initial contact with the agency explain what the WOC nurse can provide. The first contact provides enough information to interest the decision maker so he/she meets with the WOC nurse in person to further discuss the service. Information sheets about services and sample contracts are available.

- *New market:* Managed care companies, insurance providers, and HMOs are identified as other potential users of the service. These are secondary target markets.

- *Technological obsolescence:* The skills used by the WOC nurse will not become outdated. Because age is a risk factor for many of the pathologies dealt with by the WOC nurse, the aging population of Iowa obviously will continue to need these types of services. Products change rapidly and this requires someone who has the knowledge to critically evaluate them. WOC nurses are frequently the first contacts made by companies when launching new products for wound and stoma care. This allows agencies to remain on the cutting edge in determining an effective cost-beneficial treatment for their clients.

- *"No-go" issues:* Home health agencies and acute-care hospitals bill third-party payers for WOC nursing services, which enables them to recoup the money charged by UIHC. However, long-term care agencies are not able to bill third-party payers for WOC services provided in their facility. Therefore, cost of this service is seen as a barrier to a contractual agreement. If the majority of long-term care facilities do not see this as a necessary service, the WOC service will not have enough external contracts to maintain a positive cash flow.

- *Exit strategy:* If UIHC finds it necessary to terminate current contracts at the end of the contractual agreement, there will be no cost incurred at that time. Cost incurred prior to the terminations is the cost to contract with the county health agency for the 60 percent WOC nurse services.

- *Licensure-related problems:* Because of the current licensure of the UIHC WOC nurses, third-party billing for services in long-term care is not permitted. Physical therapists, who do wound care in some settings, are able to bill in long-term care, but they do not provide the range of services the WOC nurse is able to provide.

- *Timeline to maturity:* It is expected that it will take three years to adequately market this service to the primary and secondary markets. The users will require a period of time to see positive results from contracting for WOC services.

Quality Assurance/Consistency of Service

UIHC WOC nurses will remain certified and current in the practice of WOC nursing. The contracting agencies will be asked to provide a review of the services on an annual basis, which should be a mutually beneficial arrangement.

Major Events

The initial events that preceded preparation of the business plan for this service were as follows:

- June 1996: Initial contact from community hospital regarding service contract
- February 1997: Community hospital contract in effect
- June 1997: Contacted by local long-term care center to see a client; verbal agreement done for initial visit
- July 1997: Contract with local county health agency for WOC nurse at 60 percent time
- September 1997: Contacted by local long-term care center to see a client; verbal agreement done for initial visit
- September 1997: Contacted by second local long-term care center to see a client; verbal agreement done for initial visit
- October 1997: Contacted by third long-term care center to see two clients; verbal agreement done for initial visit
- October 1997: Business plan submitted, including an analysis of growth, cash flow, and breakeven (see table 3-7)
- November 1997: Contact above long-term care facilities with information regarding formal contract
- January 1998: Reopened negotiations with community hospital to continue to provide services for the hospital and home care

The proposed timeline is as follows:

- May 1998: Contact primary target markets identified with initial letter and site visit; sign contracts
- June 1998: Evaluate time used to provide external contracts; complete cost analysis to compare hiring WOC nurse or reopen negotiations with local county health agency to continue to provide WOC nurse 60 percent
- Monthly: Begin contacts with secondary target markets

TABLE 3-7. Analysis of Growth, Cash Flow, and Breakeven

Description	FY 1998	FY 1999	FY 2000	FY 2001	FY 2002
Cash inflow—signed contracts*					
Community hospital[1]	$ 7,600	$ 7,600	$ 7,828	$ 8,063	$ 8,305
Community home care[2]	348	348	358	369	380
Long-term care center[3]	2,860	3,120	3,214	3,310	3,409
Long-term care center[4]	2,080	3,120	3,214	3,310	3,409
Home care agency[5]	935	2,244	2,311	2,381	2,452
Hospice[5]	561	1,122	1,156	1,190	1,226
Long-term care center[6]	390	1,560	1,607	1,655	1,705
Subtotal—signed contracts	$14,774	$19,114	$19,687	$20,278	$20,886
Future expansion[7]					
FY 1999	$ —	$15,210	$20,280	$20,280	$20,280
FY 2000	—	—	15,210	20,280	20,280
FY 2001	—	—	—	15,210	20,280
FY 2002	—	—	—	—	15,210
Subtotal—future expansion	$ —	$15,210	$35,490	$55,770	$76,050
Total cash inflow	$14,774	$34,324	$55,177	$76,048	$96,936

72

Cash outflow*

Local health agency	$36,700	$ 37,801	$38,935	$40,103	$41,306
Malpractice insurance	300	350	350	400	400
Travel expense	1,000	1,100	1,300	1,500	1,700
Total cash outflow	$38,000	$39,251	$40,585	$42,003	$43,406
Net cash position	$(23,226)	$(4,927)	$14,592	$34,045	$53,530
Cumulative cash flow	$(23,226)	$(28,153)	$(13,561)	$20,484	$74,015

Breakeven in March of FY 2000 ◄

Recovery of investment by March of FY 2001 ◄

	Five Years	Four Years
Internal rate of return	51.2%	24.3%
Net present value @ 10%	$42,268	$9,030

Notes: *Assumes 0% increase in FY 1998-99, and 3% increase in each fiscal year thereafter
[1] Projections averaged to $87 per month.
[2] Assumes 8 months in FY 98, 2 visits @ $93.50 per visit, rate to increase by 3% after FY 99.
[3] Assumes 11 months in FY 98, 3–4 hours per month @ $65 per hour, rate to increase by 3% after FY 99.
[4] Assumes 7 months in FY 98, 1 visit @ $65 per hour, 2 hours per visit, rate to increase by 3% after FY 99.
[5] Assumes 1 visit per month @ $93.50 per visit, 6 months in FY 98, price to increase 3% after FY 99.
[6] Assumes 2–3 hours per month @ $65 per hour, 3 months in FY 98, 3% increase after FY 99.
[7] Assumed 2 new contracts per month for an addition of $260 per month.

Source: Department of Nursing and Patient Care Services, University of Iowa Hospitals and Clinics, Iowa City, IA. Prepared by Tedy Marko, Financial Analyst, Department of Nursing and Patient Care Services.

Lessons Learned

Following are some of the lessons learned in setting up a wound ostomy continence business plan:

- A major obstacle in this process has been educating nurses without a business orientation to think in business terms. Close involvement with management and financial personnel well versed in business is essential at all stages of this project.
- In the initial contracts, we did not request an evaluation on a regular basis. We also had not included a financial provision for inservice fees. Both these items have been included in the contract renewal negotiations with the community hospital and home care agency and will be included in all new and renewal contracts.
- Travel outside the county was overlooked in the initial contract with the home care agency. Because this agency was not bound by county limits, travel time became an issue. This was addressed in the contract renewal negotiations.
- As the number of external home care agency contracts increases, documentation on multiple types of forms has become an issue. Development of a standard form acceptable by all agencies will be pursued. A standard referral form used by all agencies will be developed so the consultant has access to adequate, appropriate information prior to the visit.
- Options for follow-up by the consultant were not established in the contracts. Because of financial concerns by the referring agency, a reevaluation visit is not always requested. Because of this, consultants do not always have the opportunity to evaluate recommended interventions. Negotiation of a reduced rate for follow-up visits is a possible solution to this problem.

Conclusion

This project continues to be a learning experience for the WOC nurses. Working in home care and long-term care environments is challenging for hospital-based nurses. The addition of a WOC nurse with home care experience has been invaluable. Because of the varied backgrounds of the WOC nurses, the program is able to offer a wide variety of experience to meet the needs of the external agencies.

Reference

1. Agency for Health Care Policy and Research, 1994.

4

Business Product Development

Linda L. Roman

I n today's health care environment, one of the many difficult challenges for nurse executives and entrepreneurs is that of coming to view nursing services as business products. To do this, they must be willing to place economic value on a nursing service so that it can be marketed as a viable product to the patient population that needs it.

The word "viable," as defined by Webster's dictionary, suggests such connotations as: "capable of living, capable of developing under favorable conditions, capable of being successful, or continuing to be effective."[1] One of the early lessons any business owner in the health care field learns is that without economic sustenance, no amount of good and/or effective care, product, or service will be able to continue to "live," "develop," or be "effective" in the long term. All the good intentions in the world and the caring and compassion offered by the nursing profession will not by themselves sustain a viable treatment environment. That environment can be sustained only by assigning an economic value to nursing services and obtaining that value in payment from the purchaser of those services.

This chapter focuses on the process of creating viable nursing service products. It describes a cycle of business product development based on the author's personal experience as an entrepreneur of nursing services and developer of HELP Innovations, Inc., a company designed to deliver care to homebound patients via chip technology operating over the existing telecommunications structure. The case study at the back of this chapter describes how a group practice for advanced registered nurse practitioners (ARNPs) was developed at the University of Iowa Clinical Enterprise.

IDENTIFYING THE NEED FOR SERVICES/PRODUCTS

In most problem-solving exercises, the clear identification of need is perhaps the most crucial step, but an easy process to skip over. Although drawing on the background and experience of business owners may be a good beginning in originating a new product or service, one must continually be in the process of identifying needs. Moreover, the focus on need must be free of preconceptions. The absolute goal, always, is to identify real need. Throughout the process of new product or service development, the information gathered from focusing on needs analysis will have to be reexamined again and again.

Maintaining focus is one of the most elusive, and important, skills required in planning a new product or service. Focus will come from a thorough exploration of the area in which one is working, and should result in a clear analysis of projected outcomes of the planning efforts. Thus, it should become clear which needs cannot be met and which can. The acute patient/health system, for example, has far different needs than the home environment, and strategies to meet those needs will be very different.

Focus can be achieved in a couple of ways. First, it should be narrowed to the general area in which development efforts are centered. For example, in the case of HELP Innovations, there was a perceived real need for many elderly to obtain additional nursing services. As it was, the need for additional services often led to their placement in a long-term care setting, which caused them to lose much of their independence. By focusing on this one problem, HELP came to identify many needs that applied not only to the elderly population but also to other patients preferring chronic care in the home.

Second, the identified need must be clearly articulated and defined for further evaluation. Any competent needs evaluation must address four basic questions:

1. Who are the stakeholders?
2. What are the needs of each stakeholder group?
3. What in our system/culture drives stakeholder needs?
4. How are the stakeholder needs valued?

Identifying the Stakeholders

Focus first is on the patient and then the caregivers, such as doctors, nurses, and other ancillary practitioners. Those who pay for the products and services we want to offer also must be considered, as well as various regulators. In addition, the family of the patient must be included, as well as society as a whole, represented by taxpayers, consumer advocacy groups, and the like.

Identifying Stakeholder Needs

As stakeholder needs are identified, the needs analysis process will spotlight both those that overlap groups and those that may be confined to one group. It is important to be clear about where needs align and where they do not and to plan accordingly. For example, HELP Innovations found that although payers have a need to reduce costs incurred to provide a specific range of services, these were (in 1995) inconsistent with the need of home health providers to increase revenue. In a cost-based payment environment, an increase in revenue could not be achieved by reducing costs.

By being aware of the misalignment of incentives, one can evaluate the appropriate ways to circumvent these discrepancies. In the case of HELP Innovations, two things were done. First, an assessment of the marketplace as it relates to future trends for home care reimbursement revealed that, while the misalignment existed in the current marketplace, the market trend was pushing the home care industry into a cost-sensitive posture. Second, while waiting for market conditions to create this paradigm shift, it was important to initially market the product to an industry segment more sensitive to cost savings—such as organizations at risk for overall cost of treatment. Providers who have assumed the risk for overall costs of care have the incentive to use lower-cost outpatient services when the higher-cost services can be reduced or eliminated.

Identifying the Drivers of Stakeholder Needs

Any effective development effort must evaluate whether the needs identified are basic human ones, which are permanent, or those brought about by economic, demographic, or other change that may be temporary and may or may not continue into the near future. Figure 4-1 shows needs and their status that were identified in the HELP Innovations process.

Valuing Stakeholder Needs

Finally, consideration should be given to how society values the real needs identified. Are they considered important? For example, convenience, which makes life easier for the patient, may be deemed of lower value than quality. Clearly, the needs evaluation must be customer driven, but the customer concept must include all the stakeholders in the process.

In order to completely evaluate market needs, it is useful to complete a needs analysis grid (see figure 4-2). First, it is imperative that *all* stakeholders are identified. Each different party should be listed

FIGURE 4-1.   Needs Identified in the HELP Innovations Process

Payer need to reduce cost of care	Semipermanent (economic)
Aging population	Semipermanent (change/demographic)
More support needed for a transient population	Permanent (change)
Telecommunications innovation education	Temporary (innovation/convenience)
Provider need for new data collection methods	Temporary (political/economic)
Need for social/emotional support	Permanent (human)

across the top of the grid. Use as many columns as is necessary in order to identify each group separately.

In the column below the identified stakeholder, identify the needs of that stakeholder only. This should be completed by individuals who have expertise in that particular area.

After the needs are identified, the critical process of identifying the *drivers* and assigning a *value* to each driver must be completed. A driver is an element that "controls, guides, or directs" or "supplies the motivating force" for the behavior of the stakeholder.[2] For example, three drivers for a payer group (stakeholder) could be:

a. Patient satisfaction
b. Cost of care
c. Clinical outcome of care

All three are drivers—supplying the motivating force; however, the *value* assigned to each may vary. The motivating force would be quite different if patient satisfaction is assigned a higher value than cost of care and vice versa. The conclusions should be challenged by checking the results. Will a change in the key driver change the behavior of the stakeholder group? (That is, if cost of care is reduced, will the stakeholder group increase utilization?)

PROPOSING SOLUTIONS

Nurses have the advantage of good problem-solving skills developed in response to the immediacy of patient care. A clear focus must be maintained, even in the exciting and productive opportunity for creative problem solving that exists at this point in the business product development cycle. Inherent in the creative process is the recognition that creativity is simple. Creativity is not about intelligence, but about being

FIGURE 4-2. Needs Analysis Grid

Stakeholders	1.	2.	3.	4.	5.	6.
Needs						
Drivers a.						
b.						
c.						
d.						
e.						
etc.						
Value (1–10) a.						
b.						
c.						
d.						
e.						
etc.						

open to new ways of thinking about problems, real needs, and real solutions to the problems identified.

Techniques for Generating Creative Solutions

Brainstorming is one technique for getting creative juices to flow. The goal is to create as many solutions and opportunities as possible, without getting bogged down in judging them before they are even discovered. Another technique for generating creative solutions is to participate in peripheral information seminars. For example, during the germination period when HELP Innovations' home telecare product concept was being developed, we participated in many seminars and information sessions that focused on various technological innovations in the health care and telecommunications industry. These learning opportunities informed and educated the staff. While we chose not to adopt most of those innovations, the information gathered on conditions in the marketplace, both economic and technological, had an impact on HELP's business plan.

Perceived versus Real Values

A product (or marketable service) is anything that can be bought, sold, or exchanged for a perceived value. The perceived value is generally greater than the actual combined value of the components used to create or manufacture the final product or service. While in some industries a product can be created, hold value, and be marketed simply on the basis of some kind of perceived value, the health care industry is a special case. It is especially sensitive to perceived versus real value, and this is based on the economic pressures on the industry. This is not to say that perceived value, in the form of improved overall patient lifestyle, increased patient independence, or improved patient dignity, isn't important; however, the perceived value in the patient services described above is unlikely to create as great a market value for the product as the real, or empirically supported, value.

A major factor that must not be overlooked is the value assigned to the product/service by all the various stakeholders. Value in this sense is defined in the following contexts:

- *As an amount regarded as a fair equivalent for something:* What value is placed on the product/service in comparison to other products/services similar or equivalent in nature?
- *As worth in terms of its importance to the possessor:* What is it worth to the recipient? What would users pay for this service if

they didn't have the product or service and needed it (necessary for continuing good or improving health standard) or wanted it (desired for convenience of recipient and/or others)?

- *As a standard or principle regarded as desirable or worth-while:* What is the value of the product or service in relationship to the standard established? For example, a standard of care is set that certain services should be provided in the home—the new product meets the standards and/or exceeds the standard.

Methods for Valuing the Health Care Product

With these definitions firmly in mind, we now come to the process of placing a value on the nursing care so vital to our products and services. Many methods are used in this valuing process, including focus groups, surveys, and beta testing. The process will provide valuable information that will be used in marketing the product.

Because patient needs must be met as soon as they present themselves, nurses traditionally have provided their services automatically—without thought to monetary value. Therefore, the perceived value assigned to their services is uncertain. An essential element in the development of any product/service must be the ability to demonstrate "perceived" value as well as "real" value.

Perceived value is often in the form of abstract considerations such as emotional and psychological well-being. Certainly few stakeholders would disagree that patients, families, and society as a whole assign a perceived value to nurse-delivered products and services; indeed, the nursing contribution to the health delivery system as a whole cannot be denied.

Unfortunately, an effective method of empirically demonstrating perceived value has been lacking, and efforts to create the methodology are sometimes viewed by nurses as a challenge to their value. In actuality, quite the opposite is true. In an atmosphere of increased economic pressure, the perceived value will only provide a beginning point. It must be followed by validation of the real value attributed to the products and services being developed for market. The best way to demonstrate value is through an effective standardized method of reporting key characteristics of the process and outcome. The characteristics must be key factors identified as drivers in the outcome of the process. The reporting method must be created in an efficient manner, leveraging technology to provide tools for this process so as not to unnecessarily interfere with the nursing function.

For example, nurses can use lightweight, hand-held personal computers with touch screen capability to enter data in the home. Another example is creating electronic linking systems to tie patient assessment and treatment data together into the plan of treatment.

Envisioning the Product

Armed with the information gathered from the needs evaluation, real versus perceived value, and analysis of all these factors, it is time to envision the product. However, this creative process can generate roadblocks, either real or perceived. There must be dedication to working through those roadblocks. For example, during the telehome care project's early development, representatives of a prominent telecommunications company spent an afternoon with us learning about our vision of an innovative industry that could help people by delivering health care into patient homes through the use of computers operating over the existing infrastructure. However, rather than being excited about a vision that would make vital use of the telecommunications expertise within their own industry, they were less than optimistic about the viability of the project. This could have been viewed as a roadblock if HELP had become discouraged and did not pursue other options; but believing that there were solutions to be found, we were provided an opportunity to innovate. This experience taught HELP the importance of respecting the delicate balance between the presence of real roadblocks and maintaining our persistent effort to solve problems creatively.

In addition, there must be a willingness and a dedication to continually challenge every conclusion reached in the process of creating the product. For those inexperienced in the reality of the marketplace, it is imperative to have at one's disposal at least one seasoned, respected businessperson to challenge every assumption made and each conclusion reached. At this point, a dogmatic devil's advocate or two will be invaluable, though at times frustrating.

TECHNIQUES FOR TESTING SOLUTIONS

It is vitally important to test the solutions—potential products or services—once they have been identified to determine if they truly respond to the real need identified. Testing must occur in relation to the specific needs of each stakeholder group previously identified. A testing environment must be created that will simulate the process anticipated to address each and every need, driver, and stakeholder. For example, when HELP Innovations simulated the ability of the telehealth care product to meet the social/emotional need of the patient, a concern arose regarding confidentiality and privacy. During the simulation test, confidentiality and privacy were of critical concern to the providers.

After simulation comes the actual testing on a very small scale, called alpha testing, in which the concerns and proposed solutions can be more fully explored and tested. Alpha testing should define ways to test for specific issues identified through simulation. For example, in the HELP alpha test, patients were asked in a survey document if they were comfortable regarding confidentiality and privacy. The survey instrument, developed and summarized by The Kansas University Medical Center, Information Technology Services and Research group, determined that, in fact, most patients did not feel uncomfortable about or threatened by the safeguarding of information about their care. Instead, our service gave them an increased sense of security.

Had HELP been afraid to test the issues of confidentiality and privacy, it would not have received this realistic feedback and may have failed to address the real needs perceived by the patients as stakeholders in the process. All assumptions should be challenged at this point; this is the ideal time to look for mistakes or to make improvements. Finding problems in the proposed solution is not an indication of failure, but rather an opportunity to continue the development process.

Alpha testing is essential for evaluating solution feasibility. It determines the product/service's practical ability to successfully reach the marketplace. Alpha testing is implemented on a very small scale (two to five patients or products) with the creation of prototypes of a sample product. Testing merely determines that a product or service will, in fact, do what is needed.

In the case of HELP Innovations' telecare development process, an alpha test asked if information could be assessed and accessed over a two-video connection used to conduct a nursing assessment of the patient's situation. The alpha test phase further investigated whether the connection was acceptable to the patient and palatable to the practitioner. In the case of the latter, the test explored whether practitioners were convinced that it met professional standards, that they were comfortable operating the system, and that they personally accepted the way the system worked. For HELP, this information was critical to continuing the development process in terms of commercialization, implementation, and use.

The information gained during the evolutionary needs analysis and solution proposal process should be used to make improvements and modifications to the product/service throughout the subsequent stages of business product development. The bottom line is to think about the users and beneficiaries of your products and services, both today and in the future, and nurture staged growth into maturity.

ASSESSING SOLUTION FEASIBILITY

Solution feasibility should be assessed from the following perspectives:

- *Technology:* Today's technology has an enormous impact on the feasibility of the solutions identified in the course of product/service development. At any given point, a proposed solution might be manipulated by new technology or a new use of existing technology to improve on the ways in which your product/service is produced or performed. This is called "leveraging our human resources," and the result is drastically improved productivity. Developmental cycles, which once took years, can now be accomplished in weeks.

  Moreover, it is important to stay abreast of trends in technology. For example, incredible developments are taking place in the telecommunications industry that will bring more broadband capability to the home. Many companies in this industry are working on innovations, ranging from a new copper wire technology, such as ADSL or HDSL, to the latest in satellite innovations. These technological trends vitally affect product/service development and the effective solutions that HELP has introduced. Tracking new technological trends as they become visible makes it possible to take advantage of changes as they occur.

- *Economy:* The economy also must be considered in assessing the feasibility of proposed solutions. For example, enrollment in managed health care plans has grown 350 percent in the past five years.[3] This phenomenal statistic has resulted in increased scrutiny of, and pressure on, home health care practices nationwide. Casting a keen eye toward economic trends requires watching such things as where this phenomenal growth rate is going and the nature of the congressional climate surrounding it. Also, one should watch for other inevitable trends that might develop, such as customer dissatisfaction with HMO choices and the industry's move away from cost-based payment structures to capitated, or risk-sharing, payment structures.

- *Human issues:* The realistic, human side to all this is critically important. Technology and economics take us on a roller-coaster ride into the unknown. If, for example, the need for standardized data to deliver quality outcomes is apparent but requires that health practitioners (the human side of the equation) change their treatment or caregiving behavior, a time out should be called to consider the human factor. Supporting information must be gathered and provided to practitioners when they are asked to make changes in clinical decision making. This must be planned strategically to provide for the internalization of the process.

  What drives a change in such behavior? Convenience? Relationships? Payment incentives? Know what elements are involved here so you know how your product/service fits into the scheme of things, and how it can begin to affect the behavior "drivers." Realize that changing human behavior, even for the best of reasons, takes time. Don't expect a solution to become an overnight sensation just because everyone realizes a great solution is available. The human element is crucial and requires the careful constructing of bridges from the past to the present and toward the future.

Armed with valuable information obtained through the alpha testing phase and the continuing evaluation of needs related to each of the stakeholders, an economic model must be developed to support the proposed product or service. Next comes testing on a wider scale.

Beta Testing the Product

Beta testing is the process whereby the product or service is operationalized in a real market use setting on a larger-scale population. Often, it is done in more than one type of market setting. Beta testing is an especially effective way not only to test the operational viability of the product/service on a wider scale, but also to begin to determine the important lessons of market acceptance and market value. What specific value does the market place on the product or service? How is the innovation perceived?

In addition, beta testing can be used to challenge all the assumptions made in the development process to this point, including the economic ones. For example, an assumption that it will take a nurse 20 minutes to perform a certain task, from which you have created an economic model, is now ready to be tested. Identify the critical elements for success, such as labor intensity, ease of use, and the like; then rank them in order of importance. Which elements will have the greatest effect on the success of the product? There will be surprises at this stage; some will be positive and some negative. But the ability to improve the product to meet the needs of the customer is, at this stage, extremely important.

In beta testing the telehome care concept for HELP Innovations, the following realities became apparent:

- The software database that was used during the beta phase was not reliable because of larger quantities of data than were originally expected.
- Labor intensity was lower than anticipated by five minutes.
- More technical support was needed for nurses inexperienced in the use of newer technologies.
- Certain transmission media were not universally understood and/or available.

When the discovery was made that the labor intensity statistic was better than predicted, this provided a degree of assurance in knowing that the economic model forecasted was accurate. When the training and management support needs of nurses new to the technology with which they had to work were met, the educational component of the product concept was validated. The software database was rewritten to enhance its data capture, security, and reliability with large amounts of data.

BRINGING THE PRODUCT TO MARKET

Several factors are crucial when the time comes to introduce the product to the marketplace. The following subsections discuss some of these.

Acquiring Capital

The ability to obtain capital is crucial to the ability to bring a product to market. The effectiveness of the professionals involved in creating a truly economically viable product will be the deciding factor in success versus failure. It is impossible to raise the money to market the product without selling the ideas behind the product/service. And one cannot sell the ideas without presenting scientific evidence gathered throughout the development, design, and testing phases.

Making a potential investor aware that you have used alpha and beta testing in proving or disproving previous assumptions in regard to solutions reached in the development process is crucial. So, also, is communicating the knowledge, experience, and skills of the management team and the trends that support the findings. The willingness to continue to monitor the product creation process for errors in judgments, and accurately separate fact from assumption, is crucial as well. But being aware of the importance of your staff and the role they play in product/service delivery is perhaps the most crucial of all. After all, they are at once your greatest asset and your greatest cost. Make sure that your business plan (chapter 3) has a clearly defined product and marketing and economic strategy and that the key management team is in place to implement it.

Determining Product Marketability

In a human service industry such as health care, the commercialization of the product/service is perhaps an uncomfortable function of product creation. But one must be hard-hearted enough to view the product realistically and create the proper economic model to ensure prime marketability. Thus, it is strongly advisable at this point to focus on "following the money." This means discovering the source of payment for the services and products that are being developed for the market.

For example, who benefits from the use of the product? Do they have access to the money? (In other words, can they themselves pay for the product?) If the beneficiary of the product is someone other than the one who signs the check, what benefits are there for the payer in paying? If the product is good for the patient, but the insurance company (the payer) has the power to decide whether the product/service is acceptable, things are out of sync. One must take a look at what the payer perceives as relative value. Will payment be made just to keep the patient happy? It depends.

The real source of the money, following it back to its origins, is likely to be an employer. Employers pay health benefit dollars for large groups of employees. They decide what plans will be selected and offered to their employees based on the ability of that plan to control future costs. If costs for the same coverage increase in the following year, the real beneficiary of the product/service may be a large employer group.

It is important to determine who controls the patient. While consumers generally make their own choices about the products they need, in the health care industry most patient choices about products and services are heavily influenced, if not totally directed, by others: the physician, the particular health care plan in place, those employers who choose the coverage plan, or even the government whose plans (such as social security or veterans benefit programs) are not up to the discretion of the patient.

Know, as well, who influences or directs the use of the products/services being proposed. In the case of home health, as with most sectors of the health care industry, this becomes a complex issue. The physician orders the services; social security and other programs pay or approve payment; and hospital discharge planners and social service workers assess and determine the patient's needs for follow-up care, which are reported to the physician. Carrying this a step further, the home care agency to which a case is referred becomes the "owner" of the patient, so to speak. The choice of which products and services will be used is made at this level, so the task of the developer of a new product/service is to understand that agencies get contracts and referrals based on their cost of doing business, as well as the quality, or the perceived quality, of care they give their patients. This is a "driver," so if you are to sell the agency on the benefits of the new product/service being marketed, it may help to convince those parties around them as well: the physicians, payers, and hospital planners.

Obtaining Customer Feedback

Once the product/service is finalized, it still cannot be produced, marketed, and expected to show a profit if no one will pay for it. Customer feedback is an absolute necessity, and it must occur on a regular basis so the organization marketing the product/service is constantly apprised of its usefulness to the customer. One way to obtain customer feedback is through focus groups. Whether on a formal or an informal basis, it is a well-known fact that the diversity of opinion and ideas that permeate the air as focus groups meet to assess and reassess such things as marketability make for a far more effective outcome than one opinion standing alone. With information flowing between both customers and peers, all that remains is to get that information back into the mainstream of the organization's decision-making process.

Facing the Costs of Commercialization

Most new products/services are not expected to become self-supporting for two or three years, so start-up, or seed, money is essential. However, one must never lose sight of the fact that at some point the new product must be self-sustaining. A clear plan to reach that point must be put into place, with consistent progress being made along the path to profitability. If this is not happening, corrective action must be taken immediately or the product will not survive. For example, specific expectations are set for distributing product into the market over a given period of time. If the projections do not meet those expectations, expenditures need to be reduced to correlate revenue and expenses, or new methods must be undertaken to increase market penetration quickly.

Cash is consumed at incredible speed and proportions in this phase of a new development effort. This is no place for the faint of heart or those who are too sensitive to make tough choices. The consequences may result in no cash flow to finish the partially marketed product. It will then become extremely difficult to raise further capital unless you can explain with very convincing supportive evidence the error of your previous assumptions and the steps that are in place to correct them. The credibility of your plan will be at risk. Incidentally, this truth applies equally to for-profit and not-for-profit organizations. As the term implies, not-for-profit groups may not make a profit but still must provide the revenue stream that supports all the costs of product/service development—that is, everything it took to bring the product to market and everything it will take to keep the organization viable and competitive in today's health care market.

Packaging the Product/Service

Packaging is another important aspect of marketing the product. In considering what will make the customer buy, it is essential to closely inspect the product to discover the "hooks": what it is about the product that will get the customer's attention today. These hooks should communicate that your product/service is something the customer simply cannot live without. However this is done, the lead packaging must effectively communicate the worth, or value, of the offering, and the process by which this is done must be firmly established. For example, errors may be made in starting with full packaging versus component packaging or vice versa. Sufficient flexibility in purchasing various components without allowing customization may be crucial in being able to switch to the preferred packaging. In other cases, the error may be in just the opposite form: so much flexibility is allowed that the true value of the product is diluted, and the result is customer dissatisfaction. A healthy balance must be sought so all the customer's needs are being met.

This abstract discussion of value now becomes more concrete. When the value of a new product/service is being considered, it should not necessarily be in terms of the value those offering the service place on it, but on the perceived value the customer places on it. In addition, the producer of the new product or service must carefully evaluate all the costs involved in its production to have in hand an accurate portrayal of all that has gone into bringing it to the marketplace. There is a point, in value and pricing, at which the production costs and the value attached intersect. The lower the intersect, the greater the viability of the new product/service in the marketplace and the happier the creators and financial supporters will be.

ACCEPTING PRODUCT DEVELOPMENT AS A CONTINUOUS PROCESS

After the product has been through the painstaking development process, with thorough analysis of its marketability all the way through, and it has finally connected with its customer base and is actually making money, it is is tempting to assume that the organization's goals have been met. In fact, nothing could be further from the truth. Being tied to the success of the past will make it difficult to continue the very work that created your success—the open, creative, developmental process of meeting needs in new and ever more effective ways. The process of product development is a continuous one with never an end in sight.

Rather than being intimidated by a fast-paced marketplace with a rapidly changing face that forces us all to stay on our toes, shift your thinking to view the marketplace as the source of constant challenge and opportunity: an opportunity to keep re-inventing product and identity.

In his book *Techno Trends*, Daniel Burus points out that "if it works, it's obsolete," and he goes on to beg his readers to make rapid change their best friend.[4] On the face of it, that advice can seem formidable and overwhelming. How can an organization keep the wellspring of creativity flowing endlessly on and on? The answer, of course, comes from the ever-changing, fast-paced marketplace itself. If building a strong sense of customer satisfaction and broad customer base are goals to reach for, then the opportunities to continually enhance the product/service being marketed are found in the rapidly changing conditions that surround it. Fast-paced conditions offer fast-paced solutions and ever-changing customer needs that can be studied and met. After all, if conditions change quickly, so do people. It is simply a matter of seizing the opportunity to respond. And organizations respond by producing innovative products and services to meet new needs in new ways.

CONCLUSION

Of all the industries in this country, health care is one in which new product/service development has enormous opportunities. Nursing provides great service and value to society and the health care system. The challenge is creating economically viable models of product and service for others to follow.

Meeting this challenge requires ownership of the economic needs, as well as the clinical and emotional needs, of those we serve. It requires creative problem solvers who will call upon themselves to think outside the traditional workings of the health care delivery system; people who will require of themselves and their profession that they embrace new technologies that will make it possible for us to leverage our resources. And meeting this challenge will be health professionals who have the ability to clearly define for others the economic, as well as the clinical, value of our products and services.

In these ways, we will be able to meet the needs of patients in a manner that leaves both the profession and society satisfied. The worst thing in the world would be to leave this process to the stakeholders whose only concerns are with the economics of patient care. Instead, the profession must rise to the challenge of creating clinically appropriate care models that can achieve effective clinical, functional, cost, patient, and stakeholder outcomes and that also compete effectively in the marketplace. As the nursing profession develops business products for patients and society, all stakeholders will win.

References

1. Webster's II, *New Riverside Dictionary* (New York: Berkley Books, 1984), p. 765.

2. Ibid., p. 215.

3. Health Care Financing Administration, Office of Managed Care (1997), Web site www.hcfa.gov.

4. Daniel Burus with Roger Gittines. *Techno Trends: How to Use Technology to Go Beyond Your Competition* (New York: Harper Business, a division of HarperCollins Publishers, 1993), p. 13.

CASE STUDY: DEVELOPING AN ARNP PRACTICE PLAN

Jody Kurtt, RN, MA
Martha Boysen, MA

The following case study describes the development of a product—a nursing practice plan through which advanced registered nurse practitioners in the University of Iowa Clinical Enterprise, a joint venture of the University of Iowa Hospitals and Clinics (UIHC) and the University of Iowa College of Medicine, could work more effectively with both the UIHC and the College of Medicine's faculty practice plan to provide advanced nursing services. The case study describes the process by which the practice plan was developed, focusing on describing the internal and external market forces that led to the development of the practice plan, the process through which product stakeholders participated in the development of the plan, and the challenges of responding to the sometimes conflicting needs of multiple stakeholders.

The proposed University of Iowa Clinical Enterprise Advanced Registered Nurse Practitioner (ARNP) Practice Plan is a group practice for ARNPs employed by the University of Iowa Hospitals and Clinics (UIHC) and the University of Iowa College of Medicine. The plan evolved through more than two years of work, from an initial focus on identifying the practice and value of the advanced practice nurse (APN), clinical nurse specialist, and ARNP role to the institution to a broader stance positioning APNs as a systemwide resource for the University of Iowa Clinical Enterprise.

This case study describes the development of the proposed ARNP Practice Plan of the University of Iowa Clinical Enterprise. It reviews the environment and driving forces leading to and shaping the plan's development, discusses the process and parties involved, and describes the plan itself.

Driving Forces Leading to Plan Development

The driving forces that initiated development of an ARNP practice plan at the UIHC arose during a period of significant institutional change. In 1995, the UIHC began a five-year plan of organizational restructuring and budget reduction designed to strengthen the institution's position in an increasingly competitive health care market. The resulting atmosphere of financial constraint led to significant concerns among nursing administrators and advanced practice nurses about the continued viability of the APN role. Most APNs and ARNPs did not generate revenue for their clinical services, and their salaries were included in nursing administration budgets, adding to expensive administrative/overhead costs. Concurrently, APNs at other academic health care centers and hospitals in the region were experiencing wholesale elimination in attempts to control costs. The value of APNs in improving quality and reducing costs was not clearly documented or recognized by UIHC leadership—APNs were perceived primarily as a significant cost to the institution.

The Department of Nursing's initial response to this changing institutional and health care environment focused on demonstrating the value of the APN to the UIHC by more clearly defining the role and its contributions to quality and cost management. In 1996, the UIHC Department of Nursing APN Council, one of the department's shared governance bodies, conducted three separate internal surveys of APNs in an effort to identify all aspects (direct and indirect) of the advanced practice role, patient populations served, practice settings, number of patients seen per month, and billing and reimbursement procedures. By the fall of 1996, the APN council reported its findings to the director of nursing and the Nursing Administrative Council (NAC).

Not surprisingly, the report emphasized the diversity of the advanced practice role, including direct patient care management for a variety of patient populations in both inpatient and outpatient settings; clinical resource management; patient and staff education; research and quality management; and administrative responsibilities. The report identified the need for a coordinated system within the UIHC to enhance APN billing and reimbursement, and recommended future directions for APN practice that would be essential for the viability of the role and for the department's and institution's success in a changing health care environment.

The NAC supported the report with several recommendations for action, including the development of a practice plan, establishment of an information infrastructure to support documentation of practice and to maximize opportunities for contracting and billing, internal and external marketing of APN services, and evaluation of case management needs across the continuum of care. In addition, the NAC emphasized that the establishment of APN provider billing should not be the primary focus of APN practice, because cost avoidance, cost savings, and the enhancement of quality are as, or more, important in an increasingly managed care, capitated reimbursement system.

Influence of Billing and Reimbursement Issues

Two reimbursement issues influenced the development of the ARNP practice plan: First, in 1996, the Iowa legislature passed into law a bill mandating that ARNPs must be reimbursed when performing services that, if provided by a physician, would be covered. The second issue involves the Medicare requirement for an employer-employee relationship for billing. The majority of APNs and ARNPs at the University of Iowa are hired by the hospitals and clinics; therefore, the cost of these employees is reported on the Medicare Part A cost report and their services cannot be billed to Medicare Part B. If, however, APNs and ARNPs are employees of physicians, they are generally considered to provide services "incident to" physicians and their services may be billed to Part B. Hence, the "employer-employee" relationship was not in favor of ARNPs billing or being reimbursed for services they were providing at the UIHC. The opportunity for ARNP reimbursement in Iowa and the need for establishing an employer-employee relationship between physicians and ARNPs were additional forces driving the development of the ARNP Practice Plan.

Effect on Plan Development of a Growing Demand for APN Services

While the initial impetus for the development of the plan focused on demonstrating the value of the APN role in an environment of financial constraint, the evolving institutional environment also influenced the plan's development—there was a new and growing demand for APN services, especially in the areas of clinical practice and research/quality management. The existing organizational structure, however, made it difficult to respond to this demand. Most APNs at the University of Iowa are employees of the UIHC; however, they are hired through multiple departments (for example, nursing and clinical departments such as pediatrics, obstetrics/gynecology, and psychiatry) and funded from various sources. A smaller number of APNs are employees of the College of Medicine and are supported by the College of Medicine Faculty Practice Plan or other sources. Consequently, there is no central clearinghouse for the recruitment and appointment (i.e., "credentialing") of APNs, no established process for requesting new APN resources or reassigning APN resources, no central means of establishing APN practice standards and parameters, no clear channel for communicating with ARNPs and connecting them to their professional group, and no organized system for establishing contractual agreements or billing for services. The need to coordinate APN services, resources, and practice more effectively, and to more efficiently meet the growing demand for APN services, helped shape the development of the ARNP Practice Plan.

By June 1996, the director of nursing convened a task force to address the issues related to the APN role, practice, cost, billing and reimbursement, and organizational structure at the UIHC. Chaired by the director of nursing, with membership representing all APN roles, nursing administration, finance, human resources, and the University of Iowa College of Nursing Practice Plan, the group was charged with developing the UIHC Nursing Practice Plan. The original intent of the plan was to develop a structure within the University of Iowa Clinical Enterprise that would position and provide visibility to APNs as an institutional resource, demonstrate the value of the APN role in terms of cost and quality to patient care, and establish mechanisms for billing for APN and ARNP services.

During the early phases of development, the task force focused on defining the advanced practice role. Five ARNP service categories were identified:

1. Clinical practice—direct delivery of clinical services
2. Research and quality management—applied clinical nursing research and measurement and monitoring of clinical and quality improvement outcomes
3. Consultation—providing expert knowledge and skills to customers in need of services
4. Health professional education—all aspects of health professional education, including serving as academic faculty and conducting continuing education; staff development; and orientation programs
5. Management—strategic planning, information analysis, and project management

The task force firmly believed that each of the service categories was essential in order to reflect the broad spectrum of work that APNs were involved in throughout the institution. (See figure 4-3.) Attempts to restrict the practice plan to "clinical services" did not seem appropriate or feasible since APN work often overlapped into multiple categories.

Parties Involved in Developing the Plan

For 18 months, the task force worked closely with consultants and stakeholders to develop and revise the proposed plan:

-   College of Business faculty challenged the task force to think strategically about its purpose and intent, and to identify cost drivers that had an impact on the need for APN resources. Cost drivers were established for each of the five service categories. (A cost driver is a factor that may "drive," or increase, costs; for example, increased demand for nurse practitioners would increase revenue to the plan, but would also drive costs if the demand were such that additional nurse practitioners had to be hired in order to meet it.)

FIGURE 4-3.   ARNP Practice Plan Service Categories

ARNP services may include, but are not limited to, the following:

Clinical Practice

- Evaluation of health status
- Order tests and evaluate test findings, diagnose and initiate action to facilitate implementation of the therapeutic plan of care
- Prescribe, deliver, distribute or dispense prescription drugs, devices, and medical gases utilized with the applicant's recognized nursing specialty (registration with FDEA and IA Board of Pharmacy examiners extends this authority to controlled substances)
- Perform medically delegated functions under the direction of the physician
- Interdisciplinary patient management
- History taking, general or focused
- Physical examination, either primary care or specialty
- Pain management
- Anticipatory guidance
- Counseling
- Behavioral management
- Patient consultation and/or referral
- Telephone consultation with patients or providers
- Patient and family teaching: disease process, learning facilitation, and health education
- Patient care resource management:
  —Case management
  —Clinical practice guideline use and management
  —Care coordination

Research and Quality Management

- Conduct and/or utilization of research
- Quality assurance/improvement
- Health policy monitoring
- Data collection and monitoring
- Clinical practice guideline design
- Outcome management
- Research team participation

Consultation

- Expert advice
- Health care information exchange

Health Professional Education

- Staff development and training
- Preceptor (students)
- Orientation
- Continuing education
- Academic faculty assignments

Management

- Clinical program management
- Staff supervision
- Peer review
- Administrative project management

- The Colleges of Nursing and Medicine provided information on their respective faculty practice plans, as well as input about the proposed plan in relationship to each of their plans. The financial, administrative, and physician leaders of the College of Medicine's faculty practice plan met with the director of nursing and a nursing finance representative on several occasions to provide input and options for organizational and financial structures for the ARNP practice plan in relation to the College of Medicine faculty practice plan. The College of Nursing, in the early phases of its own faculty practice plan development, provided regular updates on its plan and the potential for connections and contracting with the ARNP practice plan.
- The UIHC offices of Financial Management and Control, External Relations, and Legal Services advised the task force on financial structures and legal issues, respectively, that would strengthen the proposal and facilitate its implementation.
- The APN council received regular updates on the proposed plan, and its representatives on the task force provided essential input for the development of the ARNP service categories, as well as the plan itself.
- The Clinical Enterprise leadership—the CEO of the UIHC and the dean of the College of Medicine—provided continued support and advice as to the optimal organizational structure for the plan.

Issues That Faced the Task Force

During the course of development, many questions and challenges faced the task force, including:

- *What organizational structure would best meet the intent of the plan, maintain administrative leadership and professional ties with the Department of Nursing, and meet with the approval of the Clinical Enterprise, APN council, College of Nursing, and College of Medicine faculty practice plan?* The proposed plan is a department-like structure with accountability to the director of nursing and a board of directors. The overall administrative responsibility for the ARNP Practice Plan is vested with the director of nursing, who is also the designated director of the practice plan. The director reports to the CEO of the UIHC, is accountable to the ARNP Practice Plan board of directors, and receives assistance and advice from the ARNP Practice Plan management committee (see figure 4-4). The plan provides the legal and financial structures necessary for establishing employer-employee relationships between APNs and physicians and for billing and

FIGURE 4-4. University of Iowa Clinical Enterprise ARNP Practice Plan Table of Organization

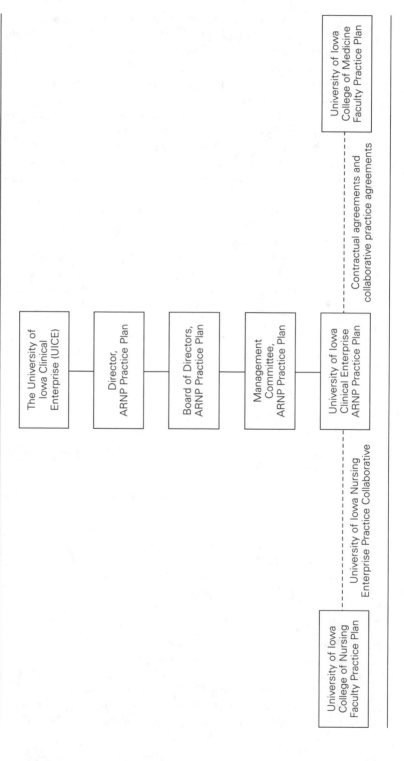

contracting for services while maintaining an organization connected to, and led by, the nursing profession.

- *How can the ARNP Practice Plan collaborate successfully with other components of the Clinical Enterprise?* A major principle identified by the Clinical Enterprise leadership, Colleges of Nursing and Medicine practice plans, and the UIHC administration that was central to the development of the ARNP Practice Plan is that the plan must not compete internally with other established Clinical Enterprise or university entities for patients, clients, or sources of support and revenue. Approval and success of the ARNP Practice Plan will depend on its ability to collaborate with all constituencies of the Clinical Enterprise (CE)—an established value of the UIHC and CE—to improve or maintain quality, enhance revenue, and/or reduce or avoid costs.

- *How can the often competing values of closed group practice and professional autonomy best be balanced?* Another complex issue that faced the task force was the Clinical Enterprise's commitment to a closed group practice within the College of Medicine faculty practice plan (i.e., physicians in the faculty practice plan may not practice outside of the plan). The Clinical Enterprise held the same expectations and standards for the ARNP Practice Plan. Balancing the requirement for a closed group practice against the ARNPs' valued academic tradition of professional autonomy brought many difficult discussions to the table. Defining the scope of ARNP practice within and outside of the plan in a way that is sensitive to both sets of values will be vital to the success of the plan with its members and with the institution as a whole.

- *Who are the members of the plan?* During the course of its work, the task force decided to implement the plan incrementally, beginning with ARNPs as its initial members. This group was most easily defined, as the institution had just completed a lengthy process of developing "collaborative practice agreements" (a process similar to physician credentialing) for ARNPs with the institution.

- *What is the appropriate financial structure for the plan?* The proposed financial structure will maintain all practice plan accounts within an agency fund of the Clinical Enterprise. At the end of each fiscal year, the plan director will authorize the transfer of unexpended income from the plan's agency fund to a designated ARNP Practice Plan trust fund. This is a multiyear revenue account within the Clinical Enterprise that provides flexibility and enables the plan to retain unexpended income from one fiscal year to the next.

Conclusion

At the time of publication, the process for approval of the proposed ARNP practice plan is uncertain due to collective bargaining contract negotiations for the tertiary health care unit, which includes ARNPs. At the conclusion of contract negotiations, the process for approving the practice plan will be determined. Final approval will be required from the University of Iowa vice president for finance and ultimate approval from the state board of regents. When the practice plan is approved, a management committee will be appointed by the director of the plan. Several significant operational issues still await resolution and implementation by the management committee.

The University of Iowa Clinical Enterprise ARNP Practice Plan will provide the structure through which advanced registered nurse practitioners, and ultimately all advanced practice nurses, will be positioned as a systemwide resource for the University of Iowa.

5

Financial Resources for Nursing Entrepreneurial Ventures

Mae Taylor Moss, MS, MSN, RN, FAAN

Opportunities abound for nurses who want to become entrepreneurs. These include creating and running different types of clinics and adult day care centers; offering consulting services; coordinating or providing educational services; and translating technology into clinical applications, including creating computerized patient records systems or networks and fashioning sophisticated case management tools.[1] Home health care agencies, a natural small business endeavor for nurses, have been identified as one of the 25 hottest businesses for the 1990s. Fueling this belief are expected high demand, excellent growth prospects, high stability, a moderate risk factor, and an average return on investment of 323 percent.[2]

Some nurses take the plunge of entrepreneurship with a safety net—they become intrapreneurs, nurse administrators or managers who develop and organize new initiatives within a corporation or medical institution. Often these enterprises are undertaken in the same mode as new start-ups outside institutions, with founders being responsible for creating business plans and marketing strategies that blend entrepreneurial practices with organizational structure.[3] These new executives are "energetic, flexible, self-directed risk takers—individuals who thrive on challenge and stimulation."[4] In other words, they have entrepreneurial spirit. Their skills, likewise, are those of entrepreneurs: leadership, assertiveness, financial acumen, management expertise, negotiation ability, and time management ability.[5,6] Furthermore, their work is outcome and performance driven: initiating new endeavors in today's health care economic environment may require proving cost effectiveness, demonstrating strategy through presenting a business plan, proving skills through expert and on-time performance, and securing funding through proposal writing or presentations.[7] Benefits for the hospital or other institution that encourages intrapreneurial initiatives include honing the hospital's competitive edge and creating a culture that enhances nursing recruitment and retention.[8]

But to put that entrepreneurial spirit to work, whether inside or outside an institution, requires money. There is no doubt that small business is a vital part of our economy, and sustaining that vitality demands not only conventional financing but the unconventional as well.[9] No one has to be a financial wizard to recognize when money is needed, but having supernatural powers could come in handy when trying to identify where to find it.[10]

This chapter focuses on raising capital to start ventures outside established organizations. In addition to explaining the types of financing available and identifying sources of financing, the chapter discusses methods of marketing to capital sources and ways to obtain start-up financing. The case study at the end of this chapter describes how the University of Pennsylvania School of Nursing took advantage of changes in federal reimbursement policies to build a model academic nursing practice.

RAISING CAPITAL: AN OVERVIEW

Entrepreneurs looking for capital need first to look in the mirror. They need to know some things about themselves and their company before they initiate contact with a funding source. For example, they must know how much money their company needs, what repayment schedule or buy-back incentive they can offer a funding source, whether their personal financial situation will inspire faith or dread in an investor, and whether pitching their company to a lender would make them soar like an eagle or run like a chicken. If they can't pay themselves or the landlord, if they don't know what CFO or CPA stand for, and if they feel more comfortable behind a desk than in front of a banker, they need to look to relatives rather than formal investors. On the other hand, if they love to pitch their company to anybody they meet, if they've had a CPA on their team for most of their business's history, and if they're making plans for raising $500,000 in capital they already budgeted with projections for earnings and going public, they're ready to have their plan checked out by an investment firm before going to the formal investor of their choice.[11]

Below are some of the types of financing that are available:

- *Seed capital:* Seed capital is funding meant to initially finance an organization through an identified pilot phase so that the feasibility of the business idea can be tested. This money may pay for research to investigate a market opportunity or it may fund the setting up of the new business.

- *Conventional financing:* For 84 percent of small- and medium-sized business loans, commercial banks are the financing option of choice.[12] These banks, too, are twice as likely to be a source for a loan, lease, or line of credit. In 1995, loans by banks to commercial and industrial clients grew 13 percent, almost doubling the rate of the previous year.
- *Bootstrap financing:* Bootstrap financing is investment capital brought into the business through the owner's own assets or those of his or her family. In 1993, less than 10 percent of small- and medium-sized businesses used relatives as a source of commercial capital, according to the Federal Reserve Board.[13] But another expert cited small business's most consistent source of capital as "private investors—Grandma and the dentist up the road."[14] Other bootstrap financing includes money generated through trade credit, factors, and customers.
- *Government programs:* The U. S. Small Business Administration (SBA) guarantees qualified loans made by banks, and, as a "last resort," in some cases offers direct financing. The definition of a small business according to the SBA appears in figure 5-1. Other federal sources include the U.S. Department of the Interior (historic preservation grants), the U.S. Department of Housing and Urban Development (for construction in targeted areas), U.S. Department of Energy (energy efficiency initiatives), the U.S. Department of Commerce Economic Development Administration (targeted to depressed areas), and the U.S. Department of Agriculture Farmers Home Administration (limited to cities of 50,000 population or less).[15] State and local governments also

FIGURE 5-1.   Small Business Administration Definition of a Small Business

What Is a Small Business?

For business loan purposes, SBA defines a small business as one that is independently owned and operated, is not dominant in its field, and which meets employment or sales standards developed by the agency. For most industries, these standards are as follows:

1. Manufacturing: Small if average employment in the preceding four calendar years did not exceed 500, including employees of any affiliates; large if average employment was more than 1,500. If employment exceeds 500, but not 1,500, SBA bases its determination on a specific size standard for the particular industry.
2. Wholesaling: Small if number of employees does not exceed 100.
3. Retailing and service: Small if annual sales or receipts are not over $3.5 to $7.5 million, depending on the industry.

Source: U.S. Small Business Administration, Washington, DC, 1996.

have programs through which loans are generated, directly or indirectly (see below).

- *Venture capital:* There are two sources of venture capital: those who are professional investors and are part of the more than 500 venture capital funds in the United States and those known as business angels, individual investors who invest at the seed capital stage or soon thereafter.

- *Alternative financing or combination financing:* Business owners can be as creative with dreaming up business financing as they are at dreaming up businesses. Lenders, too, can be creative. One business owner combined a second mortgage with lease agreements, a line of credit from a bank, and a line of credit from a supplier to create the $245,000 loan needed. His imagination was his only guide to financing.[16]

IDENTIFYING SOURCES OF FINANCING

Because bank lending is such a significant part of small business financing, it is important to examine factors affecting the bank lending industry. Janet Yellen, a governor on the Federal Reserve board, said in 1996 that the most significant factor affecting bank lending to small business was the consolidation of the banking industry, which saw a loss of about 4,000 institutions (29 percent) between 1985 and 1995. Offsetting the effects of this consolidation, according to Yellen, was the increase in banking offices (up 23 percent between 1980 and 1995), the survival of small banks in an era dominated by big banks, and the tendency of large banks acquiring small banks to continue making profitable small business loans in the pattern established by the small bank.[17]

She also pointed to credit scoring, a statistical method of evaluating the probability of defaulting based on characteristics of the loan equation, as a way banks could achieve loan standardization in the small business loan sector. This offers banks greater security in lending, something they especially value in SBA loans, which are guaranteed. Not all small businesses will qualify for loans under credit scoring, small businesses by nature being diverse and individualistic. These nonstandard loans may cost their recipients more. Overall, she reported that credit for small businesses should be becoming more liquid with a change in risk-based capital standards for banks and a lightening of regulatory burden.[18]

But bank financing is not the only option, only the most common one. The sources of financing described below represent a selection of the opportunities available. Every community's lending environment will have unique characteristics, so learning as much as possible about it will well serve any business owner seeking funding. Because most businesses are created from the owner's personal investment, we will begin with bootstrap financing. Bootstrap financing ensures that control of the company stays in the founder's hands, and every potential funding source tapped will always want to know how much personal investment matched "sweat equity." If a business owner is unwilling to risk some personal investment, other lenders may themselves be cautious about investing.[19]

Bootstrap Financing

Financing your business yourself is called *bootstrap financing* because in it the business owner is promoting and developing the business independently, without aid from outside. This is a logical extension of the early work required in starting up a business, when the cash required for early equipment and supplies needed to organize a business—but not normally required in a home—comes out of the entrepreneur's pocketbook. Sources for this money can be money on hand—personal savings, investments that can be easily converted to cash, or money from friends or relatives—or such personal extensions of credit as credit card advances, a line of credit, or a second mortgage.

Once the business gets under way, the business, rather than the owner personally, pulls itself up by its bootstraps by obtaining favorable terms or cash from suppliers, factors, or even customers, or by using assets of the business to make money. Trade credit is a method of financing supplies in the short term through an extension of the payment due date. Suppliers, for example, may agree to allow payment for materials in 60 days rather than 30 after a business has a history of doing business with them. What the business loses when operating under trade credit is the loss of any discount available from early payment and the risk of paying high late fees when cash flow problems prevent payment.

Factoring, a company's selling of debt to a collector (usually a bank) for less than the debts are worth (usually about 80 percent), is a growing method of financing.[20] A practice that is thousands of years old, factoring eases the financing or cash flow woes of small businesses, especially those unable to gain financing in conventional ways. Not surprisingly, selling accounts receivables carries a stigma because it may indicate some financial weakness that bars traditional loan acquisition; nonetheless, factoring almost doubled between 1983 and 1994 in the United States, from $33.1 billion to $57.5 billion. Some argue that the costs associated with bookkeeping, billing, and collections are enough to offset the loss of a percentage to the factor.[21]

Customers, too, may ease financial strains by writing a letter of credit. In turn, the letter of credit is passed on to a supplier as security. In rare cases, some customers may also be willing to make an up-front payment for any supplies or equipment leasing specific to their job.

Businesses can also turn assets of the operation into an income-producing holding. Businesses that own real estate can lease all or part of it to other businesses or sell it. They can also use the real estate to obtain equity loans. Furthermore, whether they lease it, sell it, or use it for a loan, they can hope for appreciating value to improve their balance sheet.

One award-winning CEO urges business owners to consider any company that has a relationship with their company as a source of alternative financing: "Look at every opportunity where you can leverage somebody else's expense to save your costs," he said.[22]

Conventional Loans from Banks

To understand bankers' thinking, business borrowers must put themselves in the shoes of the bankers. Bankers want to be sure they can recover their investment. That is why bankers generally lend against (1) assets, including buildings, equipment, and other property; (2) inventory; and/or (3) receivables. Bankers will also extend a line of credit to businesses to smooth over cash flow problems.

Ten factors influence the loan decision:[23]

1. Industry in which the business is involved
2. Economic conditions
3. Borrower's business and personal financial health
4. Quality of collateral
5. Owner's capital investment
6. Owner's experience
7. Potential for growth
8. Potential for profit
9. Business plan
10. Transaction itself

Banks vary: one may finance what another will not. Some banks demonstrate interest in particular industries.[24] The amount banks are willing to loan may also be variable.[25]

Government Assistance

The SBA guarantees conventional loans made by banks. Loans of $100,000 may be guaranteed for up to 80 percent, and loans in excess of $100,000 may be guaranteed for 75 percent. Because SBA charges for guaranteeing the loan are added to the prevailing rate, SBA loans can cost more than a conventional loan made without the guarantee. Within SBA local offices, the Service Corps of Retired Executives (SCORE), a volunteer organization more than 30 years old, provides business advising at no cost through more than 350 chapters nationwide. These offices offer guides to all aspects of appealing for loans, including a list of lenders certified by the SBA to make guaranteed loans.

State assistance may also be available. In Maryland, state economic authorities created the Maryland Small Business Development Financing Authority (MSBDFA) in 1980, an agency that has put Maryland on the minority-owned business map—one in every 11 businesses was black owned after its first seven years in operation. (The national average is one in every 32.) Its services for small and minority-owned businesses include surety bond guarantees and equity investments for business acquisitions, loan guarantees, and contract financing. The state requires MSBDFA to sustain its own annual budget through charging its customers, both businesses and banks, and generating interest and investment income. In one recent year, the agency spent about $3.5 million investing in new businesses.[26]

The Small Business Development Companies are a cooperative venture between educational institutions; private interests; and federal, state, and local governments. They provide a myriad of services, including long-term financing, to small businesses at little or no charge. Each center usually has satellite offices, often at educational institutions, and training is offered in such topics as finance, human resources, and marketing

Venture Capitalists

Venture capitalists typically invest in businesses capable of producing multimillion dollar sales within five to seven years.[27,28] Investing an estimated $2 to $3 billion in more than 2,000 businesses annually, venture capitalists are most likely to invest in a business whose potential for return is high, a characteristic often correlated with high risk. Apart from the high returns, venture capitalists are also concerned about ensuring a way to exit the operation. Otherwise, these investors may vary dramatically. Some invest in only start-ups; others invest in only well-established businesses. Some may loan as little as $50,000; others make only loans above $200,000. They may have a niche of the market they prefer. Their central interest is large businesses, and they may expect to own as much as 70 percent of the company.[29]

Angels are venture capitalists who are individuals rather than members of groups. These independent investors typically provide seed money and start-up financing, and they pump $10 billion to $20 billion annually into more than 30,000 initiatives.[30] Like larger venture capitalist funds, these angels require high growth potential in return for their investment, and also like other venture capitalists, they require that their "exit" from the venture is clearly marked (i.e., negotiations lay out whether the company will go public, whether the investor's stock will be repurchased, or other outcomes).[31]

Other Sources

The range of alternative sources of financing is broad and includes schemes such as issuing bonds, small niche financiers, and financiers who specialize in buying back orders.[32] Bonds are a cheaper means of financing, but issuing them is typically left to the largest companies. Small companies, too, have learned to take advantage of this method by creating their own large company with an aggregate of small ones called composite bonds.

Niche lenders are another source of funding. When one investment firm found in the early 1990s that small companies were being squeezed out of financing, it created an investment entity that lent only to small and medium-sized businesses.[33] Well positioned to identify investors with capital to spare, the investment firm soon had 500 loan applications to offer them and had transformed small business disaster into opportunity for the businesses, the investors, and itself. Other niche lenders may loan only to specific types of businesses. Some examples are groups that finance laundromats or cleaners, restaurants, staffing services operations, or other specific markets.[34] Others may select whom they want to fund by geographic area.[35]

Some lending operations cater to minority-owned businesses. Some local business organizations, such as Hispanic, black, or Asian chambers of commerce, can direct small minority businesses to lenders who understand their constraints. The National Bankers Association has members who focus on lending to minority-owned businesses and can help identify them across the country.[36] The federal government, including the U.S. Small Business Administration, the U.S. Commerce Department's Minority Business Development Agency, and offices concerned with small and disadvantaged business utilization within each federal agency, can offer advice about loans to minority-owned businesses.[37]

Some alternative investors specialize in financing firms with big back orders and few assets. For a fee, they finance the company's effort to meet the orders and in return receive payment directly from the client. After taking their share, the investors pass the remainder on to the small business.

MARKETING TO CAPITAL SOURCES

Having a great idea for a business is one thing; selling the idea to a capital source is something else. Different audiences may require different approaches, and appeals may have to be combined. Along with the business plan, investors may want a formal presentation in one setting and an informal one in another. Finding a capital source to which to appeal has been made easier with the World Wide Web, where many sites now offer links to commercial financing sources and others, such as governments and government agencies, who may have an impact on the transaction or be a source of funds themselves.

Business Plan

Having a well-written business plan is essential to convincing financing sources that a business idea is viable and that a thorough analysis has been made of the market and the management, financial, staffing, and other projections necessary to initiate and sustain a business. Guides for writing these plans can be obtained at the public library or at the U.S. Small Business Administration advisory offices run by SCORE. A guide to business plan writing can also be found in chapter 3 of this volume.

Called "a road map" and "an exercise in risk reduction," the business plan should be written by those in charge of an operation, and its 20 to 50 pages may be expected to take from 20 days to three to six weeks to six months to write.[38-40] Review of the business plan may be performed by a business development organization dedicated to identifying for major corporations, local governments, and other large public agencies such as school districts those businesses worthy of support.[41]

Internet

The World Wide Web also offers opportunities to learn more about finance and places to seek funding. Table 5-1 offers a list of Web sites offering corporate finance directories, small business information and news, loan guides, links between those with capital and those without, and organizations that play integral parts in the drama of small business—accountants, the Internal Revenue Service, and the federal government.

Presentations

Presentations, those formal explanations of ideas usually made before others of superior rank, are part and parcel of gaining support for a business idea. In essence, a presentation is a sales pitch for an idea. Some entrepreneurs are better suited to making presentations than others, but presentations are a reality of doing business. As was said early in this chapter, the entrepreneur needs to be enthusiastic about the idea. If he or she isn't, why should anyone else be?

TABLE 5-1. Internet Sources for Small Business Financial Information

Site	URL	Self-descriptor/Features
Corporate Finance Network	http://www.corpfinet.com	Corporate finance Web directory
Commercial Finance Online	http://cfonline.com	Business finance search engine and corporate finance news
Net Earnings: Online Loan Application	http://www.netearnings.com	Comprehensive resource for small business information and news
National Association of Credit Management	http://www.nacm.org	Hot topics in business credit
Search Scan	http://www.searchscan.com	An international clearinghouse and marketing company linking the professional investment community with companies seeking capital
American Institute of Certified Public Accountants	http://aicpa.org	Home site for 330,000 members of AICPA
Foundation for Enterprise Development	http://www.fed.org	Not-for-profit organization devoted to helping entrepreneurs and executives use equity for greater growth and revenues
Internal Revenue Service Web Site	http://www.irs.ustreas.gov	IRS forms and publications
National Association of the Self-employed	http://selfemployed.nase.org/nase	A Dow Jones Business Directory Select Site
Service Corps of Retired Executives (SCORE)	http://www.score.org	SCORE is dedicated to aiding the formation, growth, and success of small businesses nationwide.
Visa U.S.A.	http://www.visa.com/smallbiz	Tools and resources for small businesses from a SCORE partner

Adapted with permission, *Inc.*/SCORE booklet, "How to Secure Financing." Copyright 1998 by Goldhirsh Group, Inc., 38 Commercial Wharf, Boston, MA 02110.

110

Building an impressive presentation requires creating an outline, writing out the ideas, using visual aids with discretion, and practicing delivery. Creating an outline begins with identifying the main points and then organizing them into a logical sequence. Once the main points are set, ideas under each heading should be developed, using bullets (dots) at first and then numbers or letters as the thoughts are put into order. *The Chicago Manual of Style*, a university press guide to preparing material for publication, or a college grammar handbook can be helpful in making sure the outline is crafted using an appropriate sequence of letters and numbers.[42]

The presentation should be written out in a conversational tone, following the outline and keeping in mind the audience, whether a single banker or a group of several hundred. Visuals that are relevant, that move the presentation forward, and that rely on technology that poses no difficulty in routine operation can be valuable to getting a point across. In determining the presentation mode—memorization, reading, or extemporization—consider the possibility of questions disrupting the flow of the speech, the length of the speech, and the importance of eye contact and enthusiasm to the transmission of the idea. The extemporaneous method—carefully prepared but delivered without the full text in front of the speaker—allows emotion and enthusiasm to partner with ideas. Speaking off the cuff is not recommended.

START-UP FINANCING AND CASH FLOW

The cradle in which a new small business is rocked is most often financed out of the pocket of the owner. It is hard to imagine any lender financing 100 percent of a start-up, so it is a reality that even if a new business secures funding for most of its costs, a portion will still be borne by the owner. Financing the operation themselves gives new business operators majority equity and the freedom they want to operate as they please, and their investment early on encourages lenders later to follow suit. But keeping the cash flowing requires avoiding barriers in loan acquisition and equipment and work space procurement.

At start-up, bank loans may be difficult to get because banks loan on assets and beginning businesses have few assets. That is why the SBA loan program is an option for new businesses: by guaranteeing the loan, the SBA gives the banker the reassurance needed that the debt will be repaid. Selling off equity to investors who decline to manage is also a method of start-up financing. Venture capitalists, including business angels, are, unlike banks, more interested in the early stages, and they are ready when the opportunity for growth is predominant to supply early money.

Leasing equipment and space rather than buying it is another method by which business owners make their early dollars go further. The benefits are small payments; freedom from associated costs of insurance, maintenance, and repair; the option of walking away from the equipment or location at the lease's end; and the option of buying the equipment at lease's end.[43]

CONCLUSION

Though most small businesses seek financing through conventional means, a broad spectrum of other options is available. From the town square to cyberspace, a small business can find financing alternatives. And as it does, it is sustaining a vibrant pattern in the economic tapestry. As one SBA guide put it, "Small business is big business: it accounts for more than half of the private work force in the country and more than half of all sales."[44] Sustaining that contribution is a multitude of financiers, from the small business owner to multinational financial corporations.

References

1. R. L. Simpson. Technology and the Potential for Entrepreneurship, *Nursing Management* 11 (1990): 23–25.

2. Entrepreneur Media Group. *The 25 Hottest Businesses for the '90s* (Irvine, CA: Entrepreneur Media Group, 1996), p. 135.

3. K. Caravan. Nurses Use Entrepreneurship to Meet Patients' Needs, Personal Goals, *American Nurse* 28 (1996): 28.

4. P. B. Barretto and S. S. Haskell. Development of a Nurse Intrapreneurial Role: Patient Care Manager, *Nursing Economic$* 15 (1997): 264.

5. Ibid., p. 262.

6. J. Manion. The Nurse Intrapreneur: How to Innovate from Within, *American Journal of Nursing* 94 (1994): 38–42.

7. Barretto and Haskell, p. 262.

8. S. F. Hollander, K. E. Allen, and J. Mechanic. The Intrapreneurial Nursing Department: Nature and Nurture, *Nursing Economic$* 10 (1992): 5–14.

9. J. L. Yellen. Statement to the Congress, *Federal Reserve Bulletin* 82 (1996): 652–56.

10. J. A. Fraser. Show Me the Money: You Can Look for Money in All the Wrong Places, *Inc.* 19 (1997): 110–11.

11. Ibid.

12. Yellen.

13. Ibid.

14. D. L. Boroughs. Catching Cash in a Crunch, *U.S. News & World Report* 110 (1991): 60–61.

15. Entrepreneur Media Group. *The Entrepreneur's Guide to Raising Money* (Irvine, CA: Entrepreneur Media Group, 1996), pp. 55–56.

16. R. L. Russakoff. *How to Secure Financing* (Boston: Goldhirsh Group, 1998), p. 5.

17. Yellen.

18. Ibid.

19. Entrepreneur Media Group. *Raising Money*, p. 47.

20. M. Guttman. Fishing for Financing, *U.S. News & World Report* 117 (1994): 48.

21. Entrepreneur Media Group. *Managing Your Small Business* (Irvine, CA: Entrepreneur Media Group, 1996), p. 299.

22. S. Nelton. Leaving No Stone Unturned, *Nation's Business* 85 (October 1997): 46–47.

23. Russakoff, pp. 4–5.

24. Fraser, pp. 110–11.

25. Russakoff, p. 7.

26. J. A. Flagg. A Model to Grow Black Biz, *Black Enterprise* 23 (1992): 28.

27. *Inc.* Business Resources. *How to Really Start Your Own Business* (Boston: Goldhirsh Group, 1997), p. 10.

28. Entrepreneur Media Group. *Home Health Care Agency* (Irvine, CA: Entrepreneur Media Group, 1996), p. 135.

29. Ibid.

30. Entrepreneur Media Group. *Raising Money,* p. 62.

31. Ibid., p. 63.

32. Boroughs, pp. 60–61.

33. Ibid.

34. S. Nelton. Niche Lenders Hit the Target, *Nation's Business* 86 (April 1998): 44–45.

35. Entrepreneur Media Group. *Home Health Care Agency,* p. 135.

36. S. Blakely. Funding for Minority Firms, *Nation's Business* 85 (September 1997): 86.

37. Ibid.

38. W. Beech. Before Hanging Out Your Shingle . . . Create a Business Plan, *Black Enterprise* 28 (February 1997): 29.

39. A. McKeon. Writing a "Killer" Business Plan, conference presentation, Younger Technologists Forum, Atlanta (1997).

40. Russakoff, p. 15.

41. Minority Business Ventures Get Loans, Advice from HMBC, *Small Business Monthly* (March 1998): 2.

42. *The Chicago Manual of Style* (Chicago: University of Chicago Press, 1993).

43. Entrepreneur Media Group. *Managing Your Small Business,* p. 301.

44. U.S. Small Business Administration. *Borrower's Guide,* 2d ed. (Washington, DC: SBA, 1996), unnumbered p. i.

CASE STUDY: FORGING NEW PARTNERSHIPS FOR FINANCIAL DEVELOPMENT

Norma M. Lang, PhD, RN, FAAN, FRCN
Lois Evans, DNSc, RN, FAAN

The University of Pennsylvania School of Nursing capitalized on several recent major developments in academic nursing and federal reimbursement policies to build a model academic nursing practice that integrates clinical services with education and research. This model represents an important step in advancing nursing's efforts to achieve professional autonomy by offering new and financially viable ways in which the delivery of community-based nursing care can be developed, tested, and demonstrated. Ultimately, it is a test of the delivery of cost-effective care to multiple patient populations, including some of the most vulnerable.

This case study describes how the model evolved and discusses how the School of Nursing overcame its two principal challenges—securing up-front capital and integrating the practices into common reimbursement streams. It also identifies some of the lessons learned during the process.

Evolution of the Model

Academic nursing is at one of those rare moments in history when key forces—research and practice dollars together with educational and societal demand—have converged, such that by successfully integrating its tripartite mission of education, research, and practice, academic nursing can take its place as an equal partner alongside the other academic health professions. This same constellation of forces, however, is also propelling academic medicine into the community as never before in search of greater market share to sustain its own educational, research, and practice missions. In this new, highly competitive environment, embracing the new paradigm of academic nursing practice will not be for the timid. There remain the formidable tasks of retaining control of nursing's long-established community practice environments, creating acceptance in academic circles for integrating the practice component of the tripartite mission,[1,2] and finding new ways of partnering that will retain and build on newfound equity while meeting mutual goals.[3]

For more than two decades the School of Nursing has enjoyed a partnership with the Hospital of the University of Pennsylvania, and more recently the University of Pennsylvania Health System, in which standing faculty hold administrative and clinical leadership positions; in

1997, a standing faculty member was appointed chief nursing executive of the University of Pennsylvania Health System and professor and associate dean for practice, School of Nursing. In addition, during this same period faculty and staff practiced in several community-based nurse midwifery practices, a nurse-managed continence service and other community-based health promotion programs were initiated, and standing faculty in the clinician-educator track held appointments in a variety of health care institutions and agencies in the Philadelphia area.

Birth of the Penn Nursing Network

By 1993, after several additional community-based practices had been developed, Penn's nursing faculty recognized that a formal academic practice agenda was needed if the school's tripartite mission were ever to become fully integrated. The academic practices would function as a vehicle for integrating education, practice, and research, thereby providing a new level of opportunity for students, faculty, and the community. In collaboration with two different consulting firms, results from a nationwide survey to identify national standards and best practices for structuring advanced practice nursing (APN) services within university settings were implemented and then evaluated early in the development phase. The resultant umbrella organization for all the school's clinical practices is the Penn Nursing Network (PNN), formed in 1995 with a mission to do the following:

- Support integration of the education, research, and practice missions of the school
- Evolve, test, and disseminate best practice models of nursing and integrated health care services
- Provide high-quality, cost-effective, community-based health care services to diverse populations
- Provide financial resources for the school

PNN promotes a multigenerational, multidisciplinary, holistic approach to health care through the provision of essential services to clients of all ages, particularly vulnerable populations. It currently provides APN services through seven nurse-managed, community-based practices located in neighborhoods contiguous to the university. Services include primary health care across the life span to families, women's health and midwifery, mental health, and specialized gerontologic services. PNN's goal is to build substantial practice initiatives around faculty strengths as they relate to market opportunities. Notably, several niche practices serve the frail elderly where a substantial research base and educational strengths have been developed over the years. Services for other vulnerable and underserved populations, women's health/nurse midwifery services, community-based mental health and family services, and so on are based on the school's strengths in maternal-infant health services, urban health research, and its advanced practice educational programs.

All PNN practices are ambulatory; the two midwifery practices use acute-care settings only for delivery. While all are nurse managed, each PNN practice uniquely demonstrates a model of collaboration with physicians and other health care providers within several hospitals and health care systems in the Philadelphia region. PNN was one of 20 groups nationwide selected by the federal Health Resources and Services Administration in 1997[4] as an innovative model for the delivery of community-based primary health care services. In each of PNN's practices, the School of Nursing has relied on the community to help determine the specific services to be provided.

PNN is designed as an interdisciplinary model to provide Penn nursing faculty and students (baccalaureate, master's, and PhD) with APN-managed clinical sites in which to do three things:

1. Demonstrate in the "real world" the best clinical and administrative nursing practices tested through rigorous, faculty-directed research
2. Produce new research opportunities for studying and improving nursing and health care
3. Offer the best clinical teaching and learning opportunities, using new models for the twenty-first century[5-8]

A formal Office for Research in Academic Practice was opened in 1996 with university, school, and foundation support to house PNN's repository of clinical, financial, and management data. One of the greatest opportunities resulting from consolidating clinical practices under one umbrella has been the existence of this natural laboratory for developing information systems, which PNN and the school are using to measure and study outcomes of care. In this way, the practices individually and together provide opportunities for faculty to implement their research findings and continually develop new solutions to contemporary health issues. The implications of such data for nursing and for shaping health policy into the future are extraordinary.

With funding from the Josiah P. Macy, Jr., Foundation, the school has launched a new initiative to assist schools of nursing in other research-intensive environments in the development of their academic practices. Through the Penn Macy Institute to Advance Academic Nursing Practice, these schools have the greatest opportunity to develop the discipline for the twenty-first century through the integration of research, education, and practice.

Sources of Start-Up Capital

Most PNN practices were assisted during start-up with grants to Penn Nursing faculty. Private and public grants provided capital and funds for the development of the individual sites as well as for the establishment of PNN itself. The first nurse midwifery practice was begun with a surplus remaining from the previous faculty practice initiative. Some practices also received contributions from individuals and private institutions in support of their development. Funders have included the DHHS Division of Nursing, Aetna Foundation, Independence Foundation, The Pew Charitable Trusts, The Presbyterian Foundation, the Van Ameringen Foundation, William Penn Foundation, The Ralston House, The Robert Wood Johnson Foundation, and The Connelly Foundation, as well as anonymous private donors. At times, PNN's community partners have provided start-up in-kind support in the form of free rent, renovations, equipment, supplies, utilities, services, and labor. These partners have included the city of Philadelphia's Department of Recreation, the West Philadelphia Community Center, and The Ralston House, among others.

Integrating the Practices into Common Reimbursement Streams   The greatest financial challenge for most of the PNN practices has been to develop sufficient patient volumes and to secure consistent and mainstream patient care-driven reimbursement revenues before the end of grant support, since this more than anything else determines the sustainability of a practice. The historic commitment of the PNN practices to serve vulnerable patient populations in communities with long periods of underfunding for health care and social services has added to this challenge. The school's financial resources were insufficient to mount and sustain these practice initiatives independently, and while operating expenses were increasingly covered by third-party payers, a need for a bold new approach to secure capital, similar to that employed by small businesses in the free marketplace, was recognized. The impetus was provided by the opening of a PACE (Program of All-Inclusive Care for the Elderly, renamed LIFE, or Living Independently for Elders) program that required a substantial capital investment for start-up. The school decided to seek a loan or line of credit that would provide not only the necessary start-up capital for LIFE, but also sustain existing practices during their remaining start-up periods. Following a detailed analysis of its business plan for practice and exploration of several alternatives, the school secured a line of credit from the university.

With regard to patient care revenues, PNN has pursued reimbursement for nurse-managed services that had not previously been available, such as Medicaid-managed mental health services and primary care provider status in managed care organizations. The latter required

securing an exemption in the state regulations governing health maintenance organizations. Recent legislation permitting direct reimbursement for APNs under Medicare is also an important breakthrough. In
the Health Annex, the school's community-based primary health care
practice, contracts with Medicaid-managed care organizations have
been obtained; the nurse practitioners are also Medicaid and Early Peri-
odic Screening Diagnosis and Treatment providers; some fee-for-service
arrangements exist; and family planning services are reimbursed
through a satellite Family Planning Council subcontract with a community health center. Nurse midwifery services are covered by most health
plans. The Collaborative Assessment and Rehabilitation for Elders
(CARE) Program is certified as a Medicare comprehensive outpatient
rehabilitation facility (CORF), and LIFE will operate as a dual-capitated
program under Medicare and Medicaid. The Continence Program and
Gerontologic Nursing Consultation Service function primarily through
contractual arrangements with provider and other client entities.

Over the course of these early years, the proportion of revenues
from patient care versus other sources has reversed, so that income driven by patient care now accounts for the greater proportion of the operating revenues. Grant and gift revenues continue to be important,
however. It is projected that revenues will increase from just under
$500,000 in FY 1993 to over $11 million in FY 2002. (In FY 1998, the six
practices then operational generated some $2 million in total revenues.)
While such a goal is aggressive, it acknowledges the school's considerable opportunities for development at a time of great change in the
health care system and its structures. Our conservative analysis supports that PNN overall is expected to operate minimally at breakeven by
the year 2003 and may, in fact, begin to contribute to the school's
resources by that time. This will allow the school to continue to develop
and demonstrate new and innovative models of community-based care
while maintaining its mature practices.

PNN's model also helps the school to compete for alternative
sources of funding for research and development outside the typical
R01 model, including partnerships with managed care organizations and
health systems, health care equipment and supply companies, pharmaceutical companies, and the like. PNN's practices already are beginning
to serve as catalysts for generating research and education dollars for
the school, nearly $5 million since 1994. In this way, PNN provides a
research and development laboratory for the generation of research initiatives and a venue for cross-disciplinary research opportunities.

Mitigating Financial Risk   In PNN's planning stages, several risk factors were identified that might imperil its success, making the school
and ultimately the university vulnerable. Of greatest concern were any
possible financial performance risks resulting from fiscal planning

methods for specific PNN practices, insufficient School of Nursing financial reserves to absorb potential negative cash flow, the financial performance of certain current programs, and legal issues regarding billing and professional liability. A strategy to mitigate short-term and long-term risks was developed that clearly spelled out the financial position of current and proposed services as well as the steps required to create operationally efficient systems. As part of that action plan, enrollment, marketing, and cost-containment strategies were developed and a risk-reserve fund was established.

The risk reserve comprises a CARE Program cost report settlement reserve, a LIFE debt reserve based on a percentage of revenues, and a school-based debt reserve for practice that is derived from the components of the indirect rate attributed to school expenses that would be incurred regardless of the existence of practice. Excess revenues over expenses generated by any one practice are placed in a practice loan pool to be borrowed by other practices in their developmental stages. In addition, the line of credit established with the university permits planned operating shortfall during start-up of new practices.

University and School Oversight

University and School of Nursing oversight is managed at three different levels: the trustee and presidential level; an advisory group to the dean of nursing, called the Financial Oversight Group for Practice; and a standing committee of the School of Nursing's Faculty Senate. Involvement at each level has functioned to secure important resources for the emerging practices, as well as develop awareness and "ownership" among the constituencies. These oversight groups and their functions are discussed in the following subsections.

Trustee and Presidential Levels   At the University of Pennsylvania, the trustees have fiduciary responsibility for all university activities. To meet Health Care Financing Administration requirements for a governing body when the CARE program was established as a Medicare CORF, the university trustees and president officially delegated the authority to oversee the management of the CARE program to an executive committee with its own finance subcommittee. Similar models have been used for other PNN practices, such as the Health Annex and LIFE. As an example, CARE's executive committee consists of five voting and six nonvoting members. The five voting members are the dean of nursing, the dean of medicine, the president of The Ralston House (a philanthropic organization that has supported the school's practice agenda in regard to older adults), and two members of the school's board of overseers (one a university trustee) with health care and business entrepreneurial experience. The six nonvoting members are three administrators from the University of Pennsylvania Health System (representing nursing, geriatric medicine, and rehabilitation), the CARE program executive director, the School of Nursing's vice dean for finance and operations, and the University of Pennsylvania's general counsel. One of the overseer members chairs the finance subcommittee.

Financial Oversight Group for Practice The Financial Oversight Group for Practice (FOGP) serves as an advisory group to the dean of nursing regarding the academic practices. The group was created to provide financial oversight and direction to all PNN practices as a condition of the University of Pennsylvania's advancing PNN a line of credit. The finance subcommittee chair for each practice serves on the FOGP. Its members include the university's acting provost, associate vice president for finance, and executive director for budget and market analysis, as well as four members of the nursing school's board of overseers and an investment expert, all with business and health care expertise; the dean of the School of Nursing, assistant dean of finance, associate dean for practice/chief nursing executive of the University of Pennsylvania Health System, the director of academic nursing practices, the PNN group practice administrator, and the associate director for operations.

The FOGP's functions are to do the following:

- Establish, track, and review on a monthly basis performance benchmarks (financial, enrollment, and other indicators) and compare these to PNN business plans
- Monitor the debt reserve account and loan activity
- Complement the work of the existing practice finance subcommittees by providing macro analyses
- Advise PNN on the feasibility of proposed new practices and relationships
- Advise PNN on business expertise needed and potential sources
- Provide advisory input to the strategic plan as it affects practice
- Review reports to be submitted to the university leadership as required

School and PNN Governance and Management Faculty governance, including review of new practice proposals and business plans, is accomplished through a standing committee of the school's Faculty Senate. Every practice is directly linked to the standing faculty through faculty academic directors, each of whom sits on the practice committee. The academic director closely ties the practice to the academic enterprise of the school by facilitating educational opportunities and setting the research agenda. Day-to-day management of each practice is accomplished by a master clinician who serves as practice director. A director of academic nursing practices, a member of the standing faculty who reports directly to the dean, helps ensure that operating, fiscal, and quality outcomes are achieved over the entire network of practices in accordance with the school's tripartite mission.

Business Infrastructure

A lean central infrastructure, including PNN staff and resources and facilities derived from the School of Nursing and the university, supports the practices. PNN focuses its primary in-house resources on service development, service delivery, and quality management. PNN's business staff is complemented by strategic use of established services within the University of Pennsylvania and School of Nursing. These services include: human resources; payroll; purchasing; general counsel and legal contracts; technology transfer; research administration; insurance and risk management; facilities management; security, finance, and accounting; development; public relations; and management information systems.

The infrastructure for PNN includes a standing faculty member who oversees all academic nursing practices. Its business staff consists of an associate director for operations, group practice administrator, billing manager and assistant, financial analyst, information systems manager, and office administrative assistant. Larger practices (CARE, LIFE) support additional accounting, billing, and/or management staff.

Lessons Learned

As PNN completes its third formal year of operation, reflecting on "lessons learned" is timely. These include the following:

- Probably the most important lesson has been the re-formulation of the adage: "It takes a village to raise a child." In this scenario, the adage should read: It takes a lot of constituencies to grow an academic nursing practice! Continuous involvement and commitment from faculty, students, administration, and overseers at the school level have been essential, with simultaneous efforts to build bridges of understanding, ownership, and support within the university, the community, and clients and among foundations, businesses, insurers, and government.
- The critical importance of developing both business plans and strategic plans, with benchmarks and measurable outcomes, cannot be overstated.

- The effective utilization of available resources, including knowledgeable overseers, university and health system partners, and others, while building internal expertise and infrastructure, has required considerable strategizing.
- Simultaneously moving forward toward multitask/goal accomplishment has enabled fuller utilization of the strengths of the school and its old and new partners, while building a product that is still evolving and responsive to opportunities and new needs.

Conclusion

The University of Pennsylvania School of Nursing's Penn Nursing Network has dramatically increased the school's ability to achieve its tripartite mission of education, research, and practice. Developing Penn Nursing's academic nursing practice has provided a catalyst for new linkages and relationships within and outside the university, including the University of Pennsylvania Health System, that have been instrumental both in achieving financial success of the practice initiative and in helping to further raise awareness and knowledge about nursing's contributions to health care. The newly forged partnerships with key university executives and trustees and with school faculty and administrative staff, formed at a critical time in the development of PNN and its practices, have helped important internal constituencies understand the mission of a school of nursing in an Ivy League university in new ways.[9] External partnerships with foundations and community groups have helped to make it all come together. Ultimately, the school's academic practices will make important contributions to the quality of health care and the organization and costs of that care.

References

1. E. B. Rudy, N. A. Anderson, L. Dudjak, S. N. Robert, and R. A. Miler. Faculty Practice: Creating a New Culture, *Journal of Professional Nursing* 11 (1995): 78–83.

2. N. M. Lang, M. Jenkins, L. K. Evans, and D. Matthews. Administrative, Financial, and Clinical Data for an Academic Nursing Practice: A Case Study of the University of Pennsylvania School of Nursing, in *The Power of Faculty Practice* (Washington, DC: American Association of Colleges of Nursing, 1996), pp. 79–100.

3. L. K. Evans, M. Jenkins, and K. Buhler-Wilkerson. Academic Nursing Practice: Power Nursing for the 21st Century, in M. Mezey and

D. McGivern, eds., *Nurses, Nurse Practitioners* (New York: Springer, 1998).

4. D. Reed. The Development of a Community-Based Nurse-Managed Practice Network by the University of Pennsylvania School of Nursing, in *The Third National Primary Care Conference: Community-Based Academic Partnerships* (Washington, DC: Health Resources & Services Administration, 1997), pp. 129–40.

5. L. K. Evans, J. Yurkow, and E. Siegler. The CARE Program: A Nurse-Managed Collaborative Outpatient Program to Improve Function of Frail Elders, *Journal of American Geriatrics Society* 43, no. 10 (1995): 1155–60.

6. J. Yurkow, L. K. Evans, I. Cochran, and K. A. Ciesielki. Integrating Mental Health in a Nurse-Managed Rehabilitation Program for Older Adults, in A. Burgess, ed., *Advanced Practice Psychiatric Nursing* (Stamford, CT: Appleton & Lange, 1998), pp. 53–62.

7. M. Cotroneo, F. H. Outlaw, J. K. King, and J. Brince. Advanced Practice Psychiatric Mental Health Nursing in a Community-Based, Nurse-Managed Primary Care Program, *Journal of Psychosocial Nursing* 35, no. 11 (1998): 18–25.

8. M. Cotroneo, F. H. Outlaw, J. K. King, and J. Brince. Advancing Psychiatric Nursing in a Reforming Health Care System, in A. Burgess, ed., *Advanced Practice Psychiatric Nursing* (Stamford, CT: Appleton & Lange, 1998), pp. 27–40.

9. L. K. Evans. Overcoming Intra-institutional Challenges to Collaborative Practice, in E. Siegler and F. Whitney, eds., *Overcoming Barriers to Nurse-Physician Collaboration* (New York: Springer, 1994), pp. 33–42.

6

Marketing for Change

Michael R. Schreurs

Marketing is a dirty word to some health care professionals. From their viewpoint, patients aren't customers; they're objects of clinical care. I suggest to those who believe this that the external forces of competition, informed consumers, and new concepts of care will cause you, in a marketing sense, to reconsider patients as customers.

Change pervades the health care marketplace. It is brought about by every new technological development, government regulation, competitive initiative, innovative service, employment trend, and demographic shift. Marketing for change is a powerful concept that recognizes the most important forces at work in the health care marketplace—change and market need. Nurse executives who recognize and effectively work with this concept will be well positioned for the future. The concept has the potential to make nursing more attractive as a professional career choice, create new components of high-quality health care, and influence the health care marketplace in general. It requires an understanding of marketing as a powerful set of disciplines and tools that can be used to gain an advantageous position, communicate, and influence action in the nurse executive's institution, profession, and individual career path.

This chapter discusses the basic elements of an effective marketing effort:

- Dialogue
- Differentiation
- Focus
- Flexibility
- Collaboration
- Branding
- Accountability

OPENING UP DIALOGUE

Many consider marketing to be sales: creating a sales process with an offer. Some see it as advertising: reaching a targeted audience with a product or service through paid ads. Others believe it is public relations: organizing events or earning media stories about new and interesting aspects of the organization. Today, marketing is all of this and more. The total marketing experience is a part of marketing for change. However, whether you use research, public relations, sales, sales promotion, or advertising, marketing begins with dialogue.

Dialogue is basic to good communication. It involves stating explicit assumptions, reflecting, inquiring, listening, interacting, testing ideas, gaining feedback, and responding. Learning more about the market, determining needs, developing strategic responses, and building a network of support for your efforts are critical to success. Indeed, nurses are generally good at creating dialogue. They listen, ask questions, communicate with sensitivity and empathy, translate technical information into personal terms, and see the patient not only in a clinical sense, but also in the context of his or her role as a customer with a family, job, and lifestyle.

The following subsections illustrate some of the areas in which dialogue has opened up market opportunities for nurses.

Dialogue Creates Marketing Opportunities

The nursing profession's lobbying efforts contributed to President Clinton's signing a bill in 1997 that reauthorized community nursing organizations and gave nurses new opportunities as primary caregivers. The dialogue that supported direct Medicare reimbursement for nursing services was a communications effort that affected the regulatory environment and opened new and important markets for nursing. "This is a real victory for all of you," said First Lady Hillary Rodham-Clinton. "This recognizes nurses as the independent, autonomous force that you are within the health care profession.[1] The profession is now positioned opportunistically to "continue to make a difference," according to Linda Robertson of the Minnesota Nurses Association.[2] This difference could open the door to "greater developments of rural health clinics and a faster way to access care," according to Judy Collins, president of the Iowa Nurses Association.[3] Advanced practice registered nurses are able to deliver cost-effective, high-quality care to important segments of the nation's populations, including the elderly and lower-income groups in urban and rural areas. This new dialogue and resulting legislation has helped to move the profession to the next level of nursing services.

Dialogue Reveals Patient Perceptions

Consumerism is on the rise, and consumer voices have helped focus the American health care debate. Nursing has an opportunity to benefit from this activist dialogue.

Data on health outcomes are now being published for consumers to use in considering their choice of hospital, physician practice, and health plan. As customers, patients are evaluating your organization and, based on what they see and feel, they'll tell everyone they know. Research consistently shows that patients believe health care has become a profit-minded big business that is a nightmare to navigate. They see little value added from managed care. They are confused by government debate and the regulating environment; the continuum of care sounds, to them, like the latest irrelevant industry buzzword.

At the level of consumers, dialogue often consists of basic, common-sense reactions to their experiences with health care. In their contact with your facility, were they called by name? Were they treated with respect? Was the doctor running late for every appointment? Most patients are not able or qualified to judge your organization on its clinical competence, but they are able to judge it on terms they understand: on how well they are served on the phone, on the usefulness of information they receive from you, on how courteously they are treated by staff, and so on.

The experience you offer patients as customers is the touchstone of a marketing program. Therefore, you need to understand the experience fully from the patient's perspective. The old adage states, "The devil is in the details." This is true of marketing for nursing services, financial services, or fast food. Knowing every detail of the customer's experience is basic, but important. Fortunately, the customer is willing to tell you. Listen, and in the process your organization will gain marketing insight.

Dialogue as a Component of Marketing

Communication between nurse and patient is often the most meaningful of the entire health care experience. It marks the difference between a healthy experience and one that isn't. Indeed, customer satisfaction is a measurable component of marketing. In fact, many organizations now use "secret shoppers" to evaluate the customer relations standards of staff. But what about communication among the components of the health care organization itself? What is happening vertically and horizontally to effectively ensure healthy dialogue? Are the nurses treated as an important part of the team? Are they informed of management and organizational issues? Are they being asked to do more with less? Marketing for nurse executives requires dialogue with other members of the medical team as well as with the nurses delivering the care.

However, in institutions everywhere, effective dialogue is the missing ingredient in health care today. Sure, there are data: reports, meetings, memos, policies, e-mail, and so on. However, timely, relevant, effective dialogue is often missing. As a result, alternative communication channels develop—the grapevine. And chances are the quality of communication declines as the grapevine takes over, and morale suffers.

Marketing is enhanced when effective dialogue occurs between patient and nurse; among nurse, physician, and other clinical care team members; between nurse and administrative management; and between organization and community. The result is high-quality health care. Open communication is the key to high-quality communication and the secret to an effective marketing effort.

What can you do to enhance dialogue? Break down the barriers. The most common barriers to good communication are fear, distrust, lack of openness and accessibility, and dependence on old tools to deliver a message. Seize the opportunity to begin a face-to-face dialogue. This means stepping out from behind the desk, the title, and even the hospital walls. Get on the patients' turf, enter the staff's comfort zone, and open the channels of communication. Why? So you get your information straight—not the way you may think it is, but the way it really is.

One way to do this is to conduct communication audits to determine what issues, attitudes, and strategies are used to communicate with internal and external audiences. Communication audits are excellent tools for reconnecting the disconnections and improving communication and marketing to your key publics.

CREATING REAL DIFFERENTIATION

Differentiation requires identifying differences between your organization's and your competitors' service response, profiling your competitors, and positioning for impact on the minds of your patients and customers. It is a vital element of an effective marketing plan.

This is a country of people who value individualism. Therefore, the concept of individualism is a tool for effective marketing. It makes sense to tell your community or marketplace who and what you are, when, where, how, and why you are different and better than the alternatives. Differentiation is the part of marketing that will decide whether you succeed, fade into the "rest of the pack," or fail; and it is essential in today's overstimulating environment. In the minds of consumers, there are too many choices—too many companies, products, and services. In a communication sense, there is too much volume and too much noise. Just consider the number of publications you read today or the choices available through television, cable, radio, and the Internet.

They are nearly endless. The result is a perception of blandness. Everything looks the same. The need is for differentiation.

For industries or professions, differentiation is critical to providing sharper definition of services and benefits to key market segments. Today, campaigns tout the benefits of physical therapists, certified public accountants, lawyers, architects, dentists, optometrists; you name it, professions are beginning to differentiate themselves. For example, CPAs say they are more than number crunchers or green eyeshades. They are "versatile business strategists who can provide valuable insights and information top management needs to improve business performance." Their theme is "never underestimate the value of a CPA." What is your message?

What does the nursing profession do to position its members in the proper light to be seen as solutions for the future needs of health care? Choices are being made. Patients as customers are voting with their feet. They are the end user in a nearly $200 billion industry. To market effectively, a company or organization must create a position in the minds of consumers that not only communicates its own strengths, but also the weaknesses of its competitors. Marketing doesn't occur in a vacuum. It is not possible to ignore the many choices the consumer has and will have in the future. Marketing is a process that deals with distinct perceptions; develops plans, ideas, and concepts; evaluates them; then measures the outcomes.

How do you differentiate successfully? Following are some ideas:

- *Be the leader in a particular area.* It is often better to be first than to be better. Your customers remember the first organization to offer a new service or new procedure and often see the service as better.
- *Be the opposite of the leader.* Rather than emulate the recognized leader, leverage a leader's weakness or vulnerability. Perhaps the leader's size, lack of personal care, or inconvenience becomes a point of differentiation for you.
- *Own key attributes or benefits.* Caring as a selling point is already taken—by everyone. So how do you own the attributes that are important to your customer? Listen to what they actually want. Healing. Hope. New technology. Communication with and concern for their family members.
- *Market your organization as best of a smaller category or segment.* Each segment has leadership. Can your organization assume that for pediatrics, emergency care, or home health? By drawing the lines tighter, you offer the customer the ability to differentiate.
- *Focus your resources and messages on your primary targets.* Don't advertise to everyone. Don't be where the competition is, where you are one of many. Be uniquely and sharply you.

In short, you can create a competitive advantage sustainable through differentiation.

FINDING A FOCUS

Because no organization has the budget and resources to be all things to the entire marketplace, it must make choices. And it must focus its resources on those choices for effective results. Understanding what distinguishes and differentiates your organization, and focusing on it, is a strategic marketing advantage.

Marketing Priorities

In the past, service lines may have been differentiated and then matched to the consumer. In today's and tomorrow's marketplace, customers are being differentiated and then products and services are designed to meet their unique and particular needs. This is totally distinct from mass marketing.

It is also a major shift for most organizations and institutions. For years, they have focused on themselves organizationally and grown by adding services in a strategy of diversification. Both activities are flawed in terms of marketing. Marketing should focus on:

- Customers and their needs
- Ways to meet the needs with human resources
- Conveying that experience and message to a targeted customer group

The health care industry starts and ends at market need (i.e., the consumer's health). Over the years, many health care institutions have become overly focused on themselves. (It's not unique to health care; it's true of most organizational development.) Now, more than ever, the focus must switch from the institution to the individual.

The Internet as a Tool for Shaping Consumer Focus

Today, many consumers have already done their own research on the Web and are better educated and informed in their choices. And as informed consumers of your services, they have put themselves in the driver's seat. The Internet is experiencing dramatic annual growth as a personal resource for important decisions. More than a tool, it is friend and adviser. It is immediate, interactive, and measurable as a marketing aid, and it is where you will find a focused, interested audience. Following are some revealing statistics:

- Over 56 percent of the women on-line are mothers.
- Their self-perceptions include: "My family expects me to have all the answers" (73 percent) and "I consider myself Dr. Mom" (66 percent).
- The benefits include, "Makes me a smarter mom" (74 percent) and "Helps me help my children" (74 percent).
- Information on illnesses and injuries, dosages and side effects, and nutrition and weight are among the many health opportunities available on the Web.[4]

Today the educated, equipped consumer is making choices, and the responsibility of nurse executives is to recognize those needs and address those choices in a customer-focused fashion.

Nursing and the Marketing Focus

The nurse has always been the "high-touch" aspect of "high-tech and high-touch" health care. The essential qualities of caring, including listening, educating, and promoting wellness through prevention, have positioned nurses to be deliverers of patient- or customer-centered care. They understand the experiences that shape the customer's image of their services, and this allows them to focus on what concerns their potential customers. Focused marketing seeks to "burn in" the essence of a message to an appropriate target. Focused as a laser, the message should be simple, clear, direct, unique to the organization, and memorable in the marketplace. It may take a variety of delivery or media options, including:

- Direct mail with database segmentation
- Telemarketing to specific names
- Events that allow person-to-person interaction
- An Internet site, chat room, or Web ad
- A niche publication—to parents, seniors, human resources managers, and others
- Zoned newspaper for a circular or newsletter
- Television or radio health talk segment
- Outdoor billboard
- Sponsorships

STAYING FLEXIBLE

The most effective marketing organizations are responsive to opportunities. They're quick, agile, and adaptive. They know that the race is won by being able to go over, around, and through obstacles, and, if possible, bypass them altogether. A fitting metaphor for flexibility in marketing might be found in a product that has caught the imagination of the public—the flashlight with a flexible handle that allows it to be wrapped around a pipe, or whatever is available, for the task at hand. It provides focused illumination of the job with a hands-free advantage and seems to work in just about any circumstance.

Flexibility is an indispensable attribute when you are faced with current health care issues. These include:

- Increased consumer awareness and activism in health care decisions
- Research and technology driving new and better ways to address the healing process
- The changing governmental and regulatory environment and the impact on cost efficiency and opportunities for service extensions
- The often bigger, stronger, more consolidated competition
- A mobile nursing staff with more employment opportunities— across town and across the world
- Managed care and its future refinements
- Media proliferation and consumer lifestyle changes

Flexibility is necessary because no one can forecast with any confidence what future services will exist in the health care arena. Flexibility must be embraced when it comes to service. Every customer wants to be seen as a unique individual, with individual needs. Flexibility is also important when it comes to marketing. Today's winning marketing initiatives are often flexible in the following ways:

- *Uniqueness:* The organization has created a sense of uniqueness by meeting each customer's needs. There is a one-on-one emphasis in dealing with not only current needs but also lifelong needs.
- *Responsiveness, speed of delivery, and timing:* As more mergers and acquisitions occur, flexibility means being able to cut through cumbersome decision-making processes to bring new ideas to market more quickly.
- *Ability to adapt a successful idea from another service field or industry and bring it to the organization:* How many businesses have studied the Disney organization for directing a customer through a waiting process, or Nordstrom for service, or

Microsoft for product introduction? Ideas abound in other industries, which can contribute to your marketing services.

- *Flexible design for making the sale and building relationships:* Many nursing organizations promote health care through screenings and talks at senior centers, high schools, and businesses. Finding a way to open a relationship is often not a part of a strategic plan, but rather a result of being flexible enough to take advantage of opportunities as they appear.

COLLABORATING FOR NEW OPPORTUNITIES

High-quality health care requires teamwork—win-win partnerships with physicians, payers, and, most important, patients. Collaboration allows for an openness to address new, outside-the-box opportunities for you and your organization.

Finding Opportunities for Collaboration

This is an era of team building. Strategic alliances, co-branding of products and services, and new relationships are developed to take advantage of mutual opportunities.

Collaboration in a customercentric business means finding out as much as possible about the customers so that appropriate relationship services and products are considered. How can your organization collaborate with your customers? When you attempt to understand their needs in ways that support your service, opportunities will present themselves. Some might include:

- Working with a bookstore or publisher to bring more information to your customers, perhaps through your own customer magazine
- Linking up with a Web page for children, family, or senior services
- Considering transportation or delivery options for specific customer groups
- Providing stress seminars for businesses
- Making health prevention tips available via local media, or perhaps to area businesses for their employee newsletters, posters, and meetings
- Encouraging rural or urban health initiatives with nurse practitioners, clinics, and other health care professionals at the micromarket level

- Allowing customers (i.e., businesses, organizations, and individuals) to design their own health service packages
- Collaborating with the competition; for example, in the purchase of new technology or the sponsorship of a health care forum

Partnering with Others to Provide a Service Package

Collaboration requires thoroughly understanding what is needed and wanted by your customers, then providing it through a service package that is enhanced by partnering with others. This type of marketing offers benefits to provider and customer alike. It allows your organization to broaden its service portfolio, introduce new and enhanced service attributes, and gain for your customers new channels of opportunity that may not be otherwise available. Of course, collaboration requires increased planning, management, and implementation oversight that stretches the organization beyond its normal delivery pattern.

Collaboration has opened doors for major medical discoveries. Paradigms have shifted from narrow niches to profound new opportunities. And it has advanced health care to the highest level of professional recognition and market opportunity. At its best, collaboration shares the essence of what each party brings to the table in a way that dramatically changes the opportunities to make an impact on the market.

ACHIEVING BRAND RECOGNITION

Branding projects is the essence of the promise made about your service to the consumer by defining the core attributes and benefits your organization offers in a unique and meaningful way. In many respects, your brand is your future. Of all the elements that your company or institution comprises, nothing is as potentially powerful as your brand—not technology, not your facility, not your founder or leader.

Brand is communicated many ways: by the distinctive shape and color of your logo and typography; by your signage, ads, newsletter, or service; and by your customers' experiences and expectations when they are exposed to your organization's name, trademark, labels, and products or services.

Moreover, your brand is your reputation. It has a certain character and value. Consider the leading brands in the health care field: Tenet, Merit, HCA/Columbia, Merck. Each conveys different, unique attributes of that company.

Conditions for Creating Strong Brand Recognition

Branding is no easy job. In a competitive, overcrowded field where there is often little differentiation, a branding strategy is essential. Several conditions make a brand strong in the marketplace, including:

- *High customer involvement with the service:* When it comes to sickness or health, we are certainly in a category that receives a high level of interest.
- *Continuous service quality:* Whenever your market accesses your product, a consistent level of quality, service, and outcome must be available.
- *Market involvement for a sustained period of time:* You can't build a brand on a short burst of media exposure or by hosting one big event. It requires a consistent application over the months and years.
- *Positioning through advertising:* The names of the companies you know and depend on for branded products and services have invested in their identity: Hallmark, IBM, Coke, Charles Schwab. Each took a product or service from a commodity category and created value.
- *Developing a brand personality:* The brand is the real and authentic "you" as an organization or entity. The brand signifies the product or service attributes and the presentation of those to the consumer. (Many nursing organizations use brands such as "Ask a Nurse" or "First Nurse" for a customer information and service center.) Often a brand is used as a sub-brand of a hospital or group.

A brand must be trustworthy to specific people or a market segment or a niche for specific qualities. This requires integrity and consistency of delivery of your service to your market. In addition, the brand name must be relevant to customer needs. It should highlight a difference from competitors, and demonstrate something that also sends a message of quality.

The Coalition for Brand Equity has found that it takes four to six times as much effort to win a new customer as to retain an existing one.[5] So when you're able to sustain a relationship over the years and gain the advantage of word-of-mouth referral business, it is apparent that the financial impact of a brand relationship to your market is significant.

Steps toward Brand Loyalty Marketing

Branding provides "permission to buy" by establishing with the customer a trusted relationship that expectations will be met. It allows the expenditure of advertising in support of your brand or sub-brand to be considered as an investment. Its return can be measured. It has a calculable net present value. It will impact top- and bottom-line numbers, market-share return on investment, and stock value. Brand loyalty is financially measurable.

The following steps are the basis of establishing brand loyalty marketing:

1. Identify, attract, and nurture the right customers to the brand. Interestingly, a loyal customer can be up to nine times as profitable as a disinterested one.
2. Sell on quality.
3. Continue marketing to the customer after the transaction. The first purchase by a customer is only the start of brand loyalty.
4. Use the correct marketing mix. Be wary of too much promotion or short-term or nonbrand advertising.
5. Concentrate on strengthening current relationships versus going after new ones. In other words, don't forget your core loyal customers.
6. Make branding your company policy. Show all employees how to communicate your branding in everything they do.
7. Measure what matters. Use research.

EMPHASIZING ACCOUNTABILITY

Was the performance outcome measurable? Did it move the meter? How did the market respond to your efforts? You need to know these things in order to improve and continually enhance your program.

An article in the *Wall Street Journal* led with the headline "Nurses Discover the Healing Power of Customer Service."[6] Diane Kelly, a 15-year neonatal intensive-care nurse at LDS Hospital in Salt Lake City, became convinced that the medical people and the business people knew too little of each other's worlds to fix the problems of health care. A major reorganizing effort to make outpatient surgery more competitive led to what the writer called an unusual starting point in medicine: putting the customer first.

Kelly spoke of "innovation that came from people who crossed boundaries." Assisted by Joan Littes, a chief of surgical services, she looked at the whole patient experience: availability of change for the vending machines, surgeons who show up late, patient loss of control, post-op prescriptions, wheelchair availability, and more. Did they add up to a positive or negative experience?

After determining what needed to be changed, improvements were made. The results were "amazing."

- "Recovery times demonstrably shorter."
- "People went under feeling better and woke up feeling better. They left for home sooner, freeing up more capacity."
- "Today, people capacity is up more than 50 percent with zero increase in staff and square footage. Patient satisfaction is way up."

Results are what everyone wants in health care and in health care marketing.

Marketing Aimed at Improving the Patient Experience

Customer satisfaction surveys are being expanded to address the entire patient experience. At Iowa Hospitals and Health Systems, inpatient and outpatient services, emergency rooms, home health care, and physicians' offices are all being surveyed, including the billing procedures and wait times.[7] As customers are becoming more information savvy, health care organizations are as well. A new program in Minnesota is offering information to customers on the quality, service, and outcomes of its services to assist in the decision-making process. Accountability is necessary both qualitatively and quantitatively to understand, evaluate, refine, and refocus marketing efforts.

Accountability closes the loop to create a marketing process that seeks continuous improvement. Based on what you learn, improvements may be generated in patient education, referrals, your media public relations efforts, and message development. Every component of the marketing experience can be enhanced and improved with an emphasis on accountability.

Marketing as an Advocate

Marketing for change involves all the concepts presented in this chapter, but also requires a very important additional element: an involved and informed advocate for the process. This individual—a marketing director or a customer service director—must be aware of the public's desire and need to know about an organization's service to the marketplace. As an advocate for the marketing process, this individual connects marketplace and organization in a meaningful, relevant, and useful fashion. Without an advocate, marketing within an organization will be overlooked, underbudgeted, and ineffective. The person holding this position is the vital link between your organization, your customers, and your future.

CONCLUSION

Like any other industry today, health care must be marketed. The health care organization, and the nurse executives involved in providing its services, must make certain essential choices for change if the organization is to remain viable. In addition to responding to outside changes that affect health care delivery, such as new technologies or changes in government regulation, health care providers must use marketing tools and techniques to assess market need and their position with regard to meeting it—if not with current services, then with new ones.

Marketing for change essentially involves seven elements: keeping up dialogue, creating real differentiation, finding a focus, staying flexible, collaborating for new opportunities, achieving brand recognition, and emphasizing accountability. These are essential components of a successful marketing plan in the health care marketplace—today and in the future.

References

1. Connie Helmlinger. ANA Hails Passage of Medicare Reimbursement, *The American Nurse* (September/October 1997): 1.

2. Ibid.

3. Ibid., p. 13.

4. On-Line Medical Strategies, a supplement to *Advertising Age* (Spring 1998): 13A.

5. Your Brand Is Your Future, a presentation of the American Association of Advertising Agencies (1996).

6. Thomas Petzinger, Jr. Nurses Answer the Healing Power of Customer Service, *Wall Street Journal* (February 27, 1997): B1.

7. Bill Day. Not Just Patients Anymore, *The Des Moines Business Record* (March 2, 1998): 14.

7

Performance Management

Mary Anne McCrea, MS, RN, CNA, ACHE
Donnetta Webb, MA
Gerri S. Lamb, PhD, RN, FAAN

T oday, perhaps more than ever before, those of us in nursing leadership positions find ourselves asking: What are the characteristics of nurses who will be successful in the health care system of the future? What new skills will be required? How will we get our administrators, staff, and faculty ready for the twenty-first century, and what is to come?

The nursing literature is replete with descriptions of new competencies for nursing practice.[1-4] To thrive in our evolving health care delivery systems, nurses need to be knowledgeable and competent in systems thinking and strategic planning, cost accounting, project management, team building, quality improvement, and evidence-based practice. We expect that some of the key attributes that must be developed and nurtured are flexibility, creativity, and critical thinking.[5,6]

It has become our task to translate Senge's description of the "learning organization"[7] into everyday reality. We struggle to find effective and efficient ways to engage in continuous learning. Many nurses are turning to the experiences of business and industry for structures and processes to enhance and encourage learning and performance improvement. Organizations outside health care have long recognized that their employees are their most important resources. They have made significant strides in identifying, implementing, and refining strategies that reinforce and reward characteristics, like innovation and creativity, that are in demand in health care today. They invest significant dollars in employee education and training and view this as a vital part of strategic planning for success.[8]

Businesses like American Express, Wal-Mart, and Bell Atlantic have pioneered the development of integrated systems to link overall strategic goals to performance expectations of administrators and staff and to the tools used to evaluate and improve individual and team performance and outcomes. The goal of these performance management systems is to ensure accountability to customers through ongoing assessment of customer needs, appraisal of staff competency, and monitoring and evaluation of care delivery processes and outcomes.[9]

This chapter explores the application of performance management concepts to nursing practice in health care systems today. To do this, it offers a model for performance management for nursing practice.

DEFINING PERFORMANCE MANAGEMENT

Performance management is a systematic process in which organizations conduct ongoing assessments of customer needs and expectations, monitor their processes and outcomes of care delivery, and use this information to improve performance.[10] Performance management systems build on the organization's vision and strategic goals and incorporate the following:

- Goals related to meeting customer needs and expectations
- Competencies required to address customer needs and expectations
- Process-improvement methods to adjust care delivery processes to targeted outcomes

Performance management systems link customers, competencies, and continuous improvement. In mature systems of performance management, there are visible and consistent linkages among an organization's mission, goals, commitment to customers, and expectations of staff competence and performance (figure 7-1). Systems are in place to monitor quality and costs of care and to provide feedback to staff so that they may adjust processes and improve outcomes. Staff are provided with mentoring, education, and resources required for competency development and professional growth.

Few health care organizations have fully developed and integrated systems for performance management. Most commonly, organizations focus on selected components, like customer satisfaction surveys or annual staff performance appraisals. Typically, the linkages among an organization's strategic goals, development plan for staff, and quality monitoring systems are not evident to staff or customers.

The development of performance management systems holds several unique challenges for nurses. The following sections explore these challenges in terms of the three components of performance management systems: customers, competencies, and continuous improvement.

FIGURE 7-1. Performance Management Systems

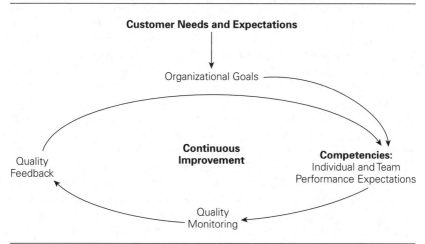

Identifying the Customers for Nursing Services

The unifying core of performance management lies in the answer to the question: Whom do we serve? Or in the business world: Who is our customer? The answer to the "customer" question gets at the very heart of why health care delivery systems exist—their goals and benchmarks for success. Only when we can agree on whom we are serving and what our goals are in relation to serving them can we talk about the skills and experience required and the systems necessary to build and reinforce skill development and application.

Today, the diverse array of customers in health care boggles the mind. First, of course, is the patient and his/her family. But to serve the patient and family, we need to work with and satisfy numerous other players, including other health care professionals, provider groups, payers and their representatives, and other departments and divisions within our own organization. Much of the discussion of new skill sets required for nursing practice is a reflection of the growing complexity of health care systems and the need to influence, collaborate, and coordinate if we are to meet the needs of patients and families.

This first step in shaping performance management systems—defining the customer(s)—is a crucial one for nurses. For many, it requires expanding their thinking about health care delivery systems and how nurses relate to each and every one of the players in health care today. It also requires that we confront the tension inherent in aligning goals related to serving patients with the quality and fiscal goals of the organizations in which we work. It means coming to grips with the reality that health care institutions are, in fact, competitive businesses, with multiple customers and significant interest in both quality and profitability. Nurses serve many more groups than patients and families, and they contribute to a much broader set of organizational outcomes than patient and family outcomes alone. In addition, changes in health care demand that nurses reevaluate what their various customers want and need. Hammer and Champy[11] suggest that health care organizations increasingly focus on the three Cs: customer focus, competition, and change. We need to recognize that with dramatic changes in technology and rapid availability of information, customers rarely need to depend on one organization alone. If one health care system does not meet their needs or expectations, they can easily switch to another. Customers drive the criteria on which organizations compete. Quality and cost benchmarks are avidly compared as organizations compete with each other in local, regional, and national markets. Unless an organization is poised and ready to support change, it will not survive.

Although there is ongoing debate about the applicability of business principles to service industries such as health care, there can be no question that today business models are profoundly shaping the structures, processes, and outcomes of health care. To develop meaningful systems that promote continuous learning for nurses, we need to be able to define "customer" in ways that are consistent with our mission as nurses and relevant to the business-oriented environments in which we seek to play out our mission.

Reaching consensus on this is not easy. There is tremendous power in the spoken and unspoken paradigms of health care, nursing, and business. Definitions of customers and beliefs about the relative importance of our goals may challenge deeply held principles and confuse and frustrate us. Payers may make one set of demands and the public another. In *Nursing into the 21st Century*, Curtin highlights this tension with a quote from Seay and Sigmond that "current public policy toward hospitals implores them to act more and more like for-profit businesses, while chiding them for not acting more like charitable organizations."[12] Our challenge is to confront this contradiction and to craft a new vision of customer that embraces our complex reality in nursing today.

In confronting contradiction and paradox, we often find that the opposite of a profound truth can be an equally profound truth. Services based on altruism, collaboration, and caring can and do coexist with services focused on profitability and competition. Opposites cannot only coexist, they can intensify each other. In *Management of the Absurd*, Farson describes scratching an itch; it is not exclusively pain or pleasure, but both at once.[13] Even though the balance can be disrupted and the pleasure of scratching can become pain, there is an absolute moment when they coexist equally. It is our challenge to create those moments when caring service and profitability coexist. It is the essential relationship between quality and cost that creates value for our diverse customers and drives the performance expectations of nurses and other health care professionals, and thus the evolution of meaningful performance management systems.

As we define the customers for nursing and our health care organizations, it is important to remember that every interaction with any member or part of our systems is interpreted as an interaction with the whole. Wheatley, in her illuminating treatise on leadership and the new science, uses the metaphor of the hologram to remind us that every part of a system contains enough information to display the whole.[14] When a customer, whether patient, family member, physician, or payer, comes in contact with anyone from the organization, he or she experiences the total organization. These moments of truth are the essence of customer service within a health care organization. If only one individual part of the organization reflects poor service, the image reflected in the organizational hologram is poor. The definition of customer is the cornerstone of performance management precisely because it defines organizational mission and reality for all members of the organization.

Patients and Families as Customers   History has defined nursing as a service profession, one that serves primarily patients and families. The public expects nurses to provide skillful and compassionate care.[15] Within our discipline, we emphasize a mission and purpose grounded in values related to caring, healing, health, and wholeness.[16] This is core to our identity as nurses.

During times of growing industrialization of health care, Curtin notes that nurses have stood firm and upheld the tenets that guide the delivery of services rather than the production of "things."[17] Most, if not all, nurses would define patients and families as their most significant customer.

For nursing, the quality of the nurse-patient relationship is a central indicator of the quality of customer service. Porter-O'Grady and Wilson assert that the relationship between patient and health care professional is core to all of health care.[18] In patient satisfaction surveys, satisfaction with nursing care tends to be highly correlated with overall satisfaction with the health care experience. In response, there is a growing body of knowledge about patient and family expectations of nurses and factors that are central to their satisfaction with nursing care. Considerable effort is being dedicated to identifying outcomes that are sensitive to nursing interventions.

Given nursing's emphasis on patient as customer, we can expect that evolving performance management systems will continue to highlight competence related to developing and maintaining effective professional relationships with patients and families. Although establishing linkages between nursing process and outcomes continues to be a significant challenge for nurse scientists, we can expect that performance management systems will increasingly focus on outcomes of shared importance to patients and nurses, including self-care skill and functional independence, in addition to the traditional clinical indicators of quality, like infection or fall rates.

Payers as Customers   The payer as customer is a concept that is central to the paradigm of business. Embedded within each organization, however big or small, is the need for resources. Cash flow, equipment, or human resources are at the heart of every enterprise. Health care payers (including insurance companies, health maintenance organizations, and federal programs like the Health Care Financing Administration that oversees the Medicare and Medicaid programs) serve as the intermediary between patient/family and the health care system. Along with providing the financial resources that allow nurses and health care professionals to offer their services, they establish regulatory parameters for acceptable processes and outcomes of care. In the growing world of managed care, payers play a powerful role in determining what services and systems will be used by people enrolled in health plans.

The reality is that nurses work in organizations that rely on contracts with payers for revenue that, in turn, is used to pay expenses. Thus, viewing the payer as customer with unique interests and goals has significant implications for the survival of any organization and its employees. If we accept that any member of an organization is representative of that organization to a customer, nurses cannot ignore their contribution to the clinical and financial outcomes that are central to payers.

Organizational Partners as Internal Customers   Nurses are rapidly learning the challenges of working in matrix and "integrated" organizations. To provide acute and chronic care across multiple service settings, nurses must team with numerous professional and functional support groups. The days of "just me and my patient" have been over for some time. All services and their outcomes are interrelated.

The growth of integrated systems and the renewal of interest in matrix structures have led to the rediscovery of the internal customer. Internal customers are individuals and departments within the organization whose work is highly connected to yours and who rely on your effort for their success. The view of nursing services as independent and isolated silos of professional care is outdated and ineffective. In truth, nurses cannot carry out their work effectively without the supports provided by physicians and numerous departments like information systems, quality management, pharmacy, or radiology. The organization's "product "of high-quality, cost-effective health care cannot be delivered if people within the organization do not treat each other as valued customers.

Point-of-service teams must rely on exquisite sensitivity to the expectations and needs of internal customers in order to function effectively and present the desired face to external customers. Team members often refer to the feeling of high interdependence as being "joined at the hip." In organizations and professions that place significant value on internal customer relationships, skills and rewards related to team performance play a prominent role in performance management systems.

Matching Competencies to Customers and Organizational Goals

The old paradigm of patient/family as the sole customer of nursing services created a focus on clinical skill for every level of the nursing organization. Clearly, these skill sets or competencies are insufficient to meet the demands facing health care today. An expanded view of customer requires new ways of thinking and new competencies.[19] A competency is the combination of knowledge, skills, and abilities integral to achieving goals associated with a position or role. Competencies are operationally translated into measurable performance required for satisfactory or exemplary performance.[20]

One of the greatest challenges is to blend clinical expertise that is core to our nursing practice with new skills and competencies borrowed from business, marketing, human resource management, and information technology. The following sections discuss the skill sets required for each of the major nursing roles: the nurse executive, the nurse manager, and nursing staff.

Competencies for the Nurse Executive Role   The nurse executive role is that of a translator of nursing care services into the language of the organization. The nurse executive is the interface among nursing, the internal organization, and the business context in which health care is marketed, evaluated, managed, and sold. She or he sets the tone and the expectations for all the nursing care services delivered within the organization. The skill set required of this helmsman role include the ability to:

- Build and articulate a shared vision statement for the organization and the nursing professionals within the organization
- Contribute to and influence the strategic plan for the organization and specify nursing's role in the plan
- Engage in strategic allocation of resources by establishing balance among customer need, market forces, and disciplinary values
- Delegate decision making close to the care delivery process
- Champion effective team performance

- Shape effective relationships and processes within a matrix structure
- Demonstrate current knowledge about national and local issues affecting professional nursing and health care delivery
- Think "outside of the box" and encourage others to be creative

Wilson challenges nurse leaders to relinquish cherished traditions in order to realign organizational structures to meet contemporary demands.[21] Today's work requires new skill sets and structures to reinforce and reward creativity and an openness to change. The design and development of performance management systems must reflect what is valued in the organization and incorporate clear expectations about the knowledge, behavior, and skill that will be rewarded.

As leaders of performance management initiatives, nurse executives set the stage and context for nursing practice in the organization. In turn, they can expect to be held accountable for the quality of their leadership, including their skills in transformative thinking, consensus building, motivational techniques, and quality improvement. Marilyn Chow, program director of The Robert Wood Johnson Foundation Executive Nurse Fellows Program, emphasizes that true leaders "build hope, direction, and meaning."[22] This is the core from which effective performance management systems operate.

Competencies for the Nurse Manager Role   The nurse manager plays a pivotal role in the evolution and maintenance of performance management systems. While the nurse executive serves as the translator between the organization and professional nursing at a systems level, the manager is responsible for the translation of mission and goals into operational practice. As the administrator closest to the staff, the nurse manager sets the stage for consistency related to organizational philosophy and daily performance.

Within transformational health care organizations, the manager role has shifted from supervisor to coach. "People performance" is the central focus.[23] In addition to the current technical skill set required for professional nursing, managers must forge a complementary skill set based on customer-focused service and people skills. They must adapt to the organizational problem-solving styles modeled by the nurse executive.

Effective managers do not attempt to control people or the environment; rather, their work is to influence the processes of care. Effective management outcomes are essential to change and to the transformation of the nursing care service as well as the entire organization.

Contemporary nurse manager competencies include:

- Team building
- Systems thinking and complex problem solving

- Change and conflict management
- Knowledge and experience of facilitating quality improvement processes
- Effective use of motivational strategies
- Mentoring
- Evaluation and interpretation of quality information

Current literature suggests that changes in the health care system have affected middle managers more than any other organizational role.[24,25] Indeed, managers set the daily pace for performance in integrated, customer-oriented systems. While many middle managers have risen through the ranks based on clinical expertise, they now find themselves at the hub of performance management systems with responsibilities for developing, nurturing, and evaluating new and/or redesigned systems of care, mentoring their staff, and making complex decisions about resource allocation.

Competencies for Nursing Staff   The clinical staff are the ultimate translators of the organization's mission and goals. It is in the day-to-day work with patients, payers, and professional colleagues that quality and financial goals are achieved. Staff members provide the central products of the health care organization. They work daily with core processes and are the most likely individuals to identify process problems and opportunities for improvement. As noted above, one of the greatest challenges for the nurse executive and the nurse manager is to craft an environment in which staff are empowered to perform at their optimum level and are actively engaged in seeking new and better ways to improve the quality of care.

Expectations of staff continue to evolve. In addition to clinical expertise, effective operational performance requires a broader systems perspective and critical analysis of clinical processes and outcomes. Staff members are asked to understand their work in the context of larger systems goals and processes. They work in complex matrix arrangements where all operational functions are linked. Effective team performance is expected and increasingly used as a major criterion for allocating rewards. The focus on results, rather than activity, demands active analysis of daily work patterns and their impact on desired outcomes.[26]

Effective performance management systems align the vision, goals, and performance indicators of administrators and staff. They tap into the power of shared commitment and passion for excellence.[27] For nursing, these systems must evolve from a broadened view of customer needs and expectations and with recognition of the expanded knowledge, skills, and abilities required to achieve desired quality and cost outcomes. Ultimately, integrated performance management systems bring together and refine the match between organizational processes, including systems for competency assessment and improvement, quality monitoring and improvement, and outcomes of care.

Developing Systems for Continuous Improvement

The third component of performance management systems incorporates structures and processes for continuous quality improvement. Based on clear articulation of the organization's strategic goals and the requisite skills and competencies associated with them, quality improvement systems are set in place to monitor performance and provide feedback to customers and staff.

Most health care organizations have developed systems to track and report selected quality and cost outcomes and patient satisfaction. Most commonly, outcomes are chosen according to customer expectations, organizational priorities, and/or credentialing requirements. Clinical quality indicators may include both general health outcome measures (health status, functional performance, and infection and fall rates, for example) and condition-specific indicators (cardiac mortality, diabetic control). Financial outcomes typically focus on cost and utilization of services. Increasingly, organizations are choosing to measure quality outcomes using standardized instruments and measures that may be benchmarked against national or regional data. In some cases, the use of specific outcome instruments is mandated by regulatory agencies.

Organizations practicing continuous quality improvement evaluate trends in their outcome data and look for significant variation between expected and actual outcomes. Variation serves as a trigger for process improvement activities. For example, higher-than-expected readmission rates for discharged patients with congestive heart failure might lead to an evaluation of discharge planning and referral processes. Increased infection rates could lead to analysis of post-surgical wound care procedures.

Participation in quality improvement activities requires that nurses:

- Understand the rationale for selection of system, department, and unit outcomes and the relationship between outcomes at each of these levels
- Contribute to the selection of outcomes based on priorities for nursing care delivery
- Be able to interpret reports of outcome data
- Actively look for opportunities to improve practice
- Critically analyze nursing's contribution to global and condition-specific outcomes
- Work collaboratively with other disciplines to improve clinical processes

Although the basic principles of quality improvement are well developed, their application and significance to nursing practice continue to evolve. Selection, measurement, and evaluation of clinical and cost outcomes have been the focus of considerable attention in nursing. There is particular interest in identifying outcomes that are sensitive to nursing care and interventions. It is very important that nurses participating in quality improvement make a strong case for the inclusion of these nursing-sensitive outcomes in quality monitoring and reporting activities. This is essential for refinement of nursing care in health care organizations and recognition of nursing's vital contribution to quality and cost outcomes.

DEVELOPING A PERFORMANCE MANAGEMENT MODEL FOR NURSING SYSTEMS

Traditional approaches to performance management are no longer adequate to aid the nurse executive in transforming the organization. Approaches that consist solely of annual performance appraisals and quarterly patient satisfaction surveys cannot substitute for models that clearly and coherently link an organization's goals, commitment to customers, expectations about management and staff competence, and quality improvement activities. Each of these components must be brought together in a flexible model that serves as the key strategic tool to manage the human performance of an organization. This model considers stakeholders, partners, customers, and employees and enables the nurse executive to reengineer and build new nursing organizations.

Developing a performance management model begins with an analysis on three different levels within an organization (figure 7-2):

1. The strategic or organizational level
2. The operational or department level
3. The individual employee level

At each level, goals, competencies, and quality measures are defined based on a common view of customer needs and expectations and the characteristics of the environment in which the organization functions.

Strategic Level

Goals and priorities established at the strategic level influence the formulation of goals at each successive level. Department and individual

FIGURE 7-2.   Integrated Performance Management

- Needs of target population (customer)
- Marketplace demands and competition
- Regulatory agencies
- Partner/provider relationships

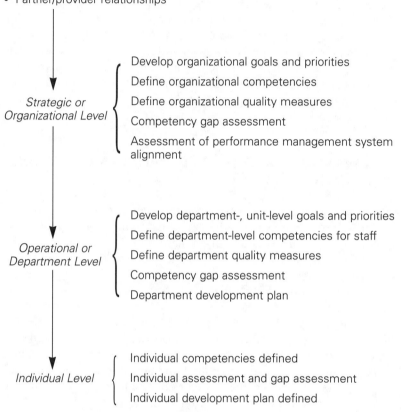

Strategic or Organizational Level
{
Develop organizational goals and priorities

Define organizational competencies

Define organizational quality measures

Competency gap assessment

Assessment of performance management system alignment
}

Operational or Department Level
{
Develop department-, unit-level goals and priorities

Define department-level competencies for staff

Define department quality measures

Competency gap assessment

Department development plan
}

Individual Level
{
Individual competencies defined

Individual assessment and gap assessment

Individual development plan defined
}

goals complement strategic goals and serve as the basis for determining level-specific competencies and quality improvement activities.

Goals   The nurse executive works closely with the institution's executive team to formulate goals that reflect the organization's vision, including its mission, values, customer needs, competitive environment, stakeholders, and partners. These goals translate the mission into concrete terms. As stated earlier, the nurse executive is a translator of nursing care service into the language of the organization and vice versa. At the strategic executive level of the organization, he or she must integrate the language of marketing and finance with a strong stand on advocacy for holistic, high-quality care.

As an example, let's assume that the organization has identified a major strategic goal of implementing a cardiovascular product line. The envisioned product line includes both acute and chronic care services for individuals with cardiovascular conditions. The executive board has determined that there is market demand for these cardiovascular services, that they will be sufficiently profitable, and that physician partners and payers support the product line. A major role for the nurse executive is to communicate the value of developing the product line in terms of the organization's mission and future. Using the language and tools of marketing and finance, she or he creates a context in which professional staff can understand and support the new strategic direction and the changes that accompany it. Ideally, the initiation of a new product line is shared with staff as an important opportunity to expand and refine current care delivery processes and to partner with key customer groups in new ways. As the new cardiovascular product line emerges, the nurse executive guides the vision of how services will be delivered. The strategic goals of the organization must be translated into a practice model or framework that is consistent with professional values and practice standards. The practice model that supports the cardiovascular product line drives the definition and scope of competencies for staff at successive levels of the organization.

Competencies   Two steps are involved in establishing competencies at the strategic level: defining the competencies at all levels of the organization and then establishing systems to integrate them.

Defining competencies: Defining competencies must begin at the strategic level of the organization if the organization is to bring together mission, goals, customer needs, performance, and outcomes. Traditionally, organizations overlook the importance of formulating a strategic/ organizational vision of competence and define competencies at the operational level only. Omitting this crucial step leaves the performance management system without an anchor to guide it.

Definitions of competency at the strategic level focus on the needs of the customer and the broad knowledge and skill sets that will enable the organization to achieve its preferred future. After global competencies, like communication or team building, are defined, they must be refined and specified to include quality indicators or measurement criteria that will be used to evaluate success. At the strategic level, competency development is driven by the "big picture" vision of the organization. This is where the translation to operational performance begins.

In the example of the cardiovascular product line discussed earlier, the nurse executive might ask: What knowledge, skills, and abilities will be integral to developing a cardiovascular product line that delivers high-quality, cost-effective patient care, establishes successful relationships with providers and partners, benefits the community, and is profitable for the organization? Identification of necessary competencies cascades from competencies required at the executive level to competencies required at each level of the organization; that is, the nurse executive's role in the design and implementation of the cardiovascular product lines requires knowledge and skill in strategic planning and budget analysis, successful performance of the cardiovascular product line manager demands excellent project management and team-building skills, and so on through each level of the organization. At each step, essential competencies are defined, linked to other levels of the organization, and translated into quality measures that will permit ongoing evaluation and improvement.

Establishing systems to integrate aligned competencies: As the executive team shapes the strategic plan of the organization and determines needed competencies, an effective structure must be in place to ensure that each part of the performance management system is present and integrated. Definitions of competencies must be translated into systems that use this work as the basis for staff selection and recruitment, education and training priorities, and evaluation and rewards (figure 7-3). At a minimum, the nurse executive, the human resources division, and the areas of the organization responsible for coordinating quality improvement must come together for optimal performance management.

Referring again to the example of the cardiovascular product line, the nurse executive has now proceeded through an initial assessment of the knowledge, skills, and abilities integral to the success of the product line. Quality improvement and key business indicators have been identified, including quality-of-care indicators, measures of customer satisfaction, and profitability. A gap analysis is then undertaken to determine the difference between staff competencies required for a successful

**FIGURE 7-3.   Competency-Based Performance
                Management Systems**

Competencies Defined

→ Goal/performance expectation-setting process

→ Selection processes: recruitment, selection, promotion, outplacement

→ Training and development, career planning opportunities

→ Performance appraisal

→ Compensation, reward, recognition

product line and those that exist in the current staff or the employment market. The gap analysis provides the strategic direction and guidelines for the recruitment and selection of staff for the cardiovascular product line and for ongoing education of product-line staff.

If the nurse executive determines, for example, that customer-service and teamwork competencies are integral to the success of the product line, he or she will have to work closely with the director of human resources to ensure that the current performance management system is aligned with these expectations. Together, they will evaluate whether the current performance management tools place the appropriate emphasis on measurement and evaluation of teamwork and customer service and whether reward systems are commensurate with the expected competencies. Consistency of expectations and rewards sends a strong message to employees about management's commitment to the organization's values and goals. As mission, values, goals, competencies, measurement systems, and incentives are aligned, organizational leadership, and particularly the nurse executive, are seen as "walking the talk."

Clearly, the nurse executive and the director of human resources will have to develop a competency-based performance management structure. The competency-based components of the performance management system need to be internally consistent and aligned with strategic goals and quality outcomes. Mission and goals drive performance expectations which, in turn, shape processes for staff selection, advancement, education, compensation, and rewards.

Competencies essential for successful performance are incorporated into job descriptions and drive the staff selection process. Recruiters are prepared to focus on knowledge and skills that are core to achievement of quality outcomes. The staffing function, while often hurried or overlooked, is one of the most important components of performance management since it shapes the flow of needed talent and skill into, through, and out of the organization. Training, education, career planning, coaching, and mentoring functions all support competence development and improvement. Reward systems reinforce the value placed on successful performance, required knowledge and skill, and performance improvement.

The nurse executive and the director of human resources also must collaborate to continuously improve the performance management system. They must be constantly vigilant to ensure obvious consistency between the organizational mission, goals, and priorities and the system that operationally defines what is valued and rewarded in the organization. An example of a common mismatch in many business organizations is when the organization's policy "is to encourage risk taking and innovation, but the rewards are given for economic results and meeting business goals."[28] Beckhard and Pritchard note further that "[t]here is probably no single action management can take that will affect credibility more than making sure that the organization's strategies, policies, and pay, as well as more informal rewards and signals, are in conformity with each other."[29]

Department and Individual Levels

After global competencies are defined at the strategic level, they can be used as the template for competency development for departments and individuals within the organization. Consistent with the performance management process at the strategic level, competencies at the department and individual levels need to drive staff recruitment and selection and education and reward systems. Each level must be consistent with the others for synergy to occur within the organization.

Goals and Competencies   The strategic level system need not be finalized before moving to the department and individual levels. Refinement between the levels of the organization is an interactive and iterative process that requires full participation of the organization. With coaching from the nurse executive, nursing managers at the department or operational level can assume significant responsibility for defining and evaluating competencies at the operational level.

Returning to our example, as the nurse executive and nurse managers design the cardiovascular product line in collaboration with key customers and internal partners, the nurse executive emphasizes the role of mission, goals, and strategic plan in its development. Competencies at the strategic level are operationally translated at the departmental level. Together, the nurse executive and the product-line manager define management and staff competencies and quality indicators. Current gaps in competency are assessed and education programs implemented.

Throughout this process, the nurse executive reinforces the connection among mission, customer need and expectations, competencies, and continuous improvement. Core competencies, like customer focus and team relationship, are emphasized, role modeled, and evaluated at every level of the organization. Systems are put into place to ensure that managers and staff participate in, refine, and benefit from an integrated performance management system.

As stated earlier, the most important focus of the performance management system and its components is achievement of outcomes based on customer expectations. As competencies are defined at the departmental and individual levels, outcomes also are specified for each level. The match between an organization's internal processes and its external demands is referred to as its organizational capability.

> Organizational capability is the ability of a firm to manage people to gain a competitive advantage. This method focuses internal organizational

processes and systems on meeting customers' needs and ensures that the skills and efforts of employees are directed toward achieving the goals of the organization as a whole. In this way, employees become a critical résource for competitiveness that will sustain itself over time.[30]

To be maximally effective, organizations must continually generate competencies in a dynamic and ongoing process. Thus, the performance management system must also be flexible and easy to modify with the development and definition of new competencies. Given the fast pace of change and the dynamic nature of the health care environment, this is essential for the organization to maintain its competitive advantage.

CONCLUSION

An integrated, flexible performance management system is key to the transformation of nursing practice and the organization as a whole. The nurse executive's main function in this endeavor is to translate organizational needs into competencies, to communicate and assist in the translation of these strategic competencies to a department and individual level, and then to communicate the achievement of standards and feedback up through the organization to the strategic level to begin the process again. This process must not be dependent on the traditional annual performance appraisal and goal-setting process, but must occur "just in time" of organizational need.

The entire communication process—from the organizational level through the individual level and back to the organizational level—is defined and driven by quality criteria, which is how one measures the fulfillment of customer needs and expectations. The beginning, middle, and end of the entire performance management process is driven by and for customer need and expectations. A performance management system is a tool for managing the performance of the organization, departments, and individuals to ensure that, ultimately, high-quality, cost-effective care is delivered to meet the needs and the satisfaction of the customer.

References

1. D. J. Pesut. Twenty-first Century Learning, *Nursing Outlook* 46, no. 1 (1998): 37.

2. T. Porter-O'Grady and C. K. Wilson. *The Leadership Revolution in Health Care: Altering Systems, Changing Behaviors* (Gaithersburg, MD: Aspen Publishers, 1995).

3. T. R. Misener and others. National Delphi Study to Determine Competencies for Nursing Leadership in Public Health, *Image: Journal of Nursing Scholarship* 29, no. 1 (1997): 47–51.

4. J. E. Ridenour. Nurse Leadership Competencies for the 21st Century. *Seminar for Nurse Managers* 4, no. 2 (1996): 93–97.

5. M. Fralic. The New Era Nurse Executive: Centerpiece Characteristics, *JONA* 23, no. 1 (1993): 7–8.

6. K. Kerfoot. The New Nursing Leader for the New World Order of Health Care, *Nursing Economic$* 14, no. 4 (1996): 239–40.

7. P. M. Senge. *The Fifth Discipline: The Art and Practice of the Learning Organization* (New York: Currency Doubleday, 1990).

8. M. A. Verespej. Lessons from the Best. *Industry Week* 247, no. 4 (1998): 28–35.

9. C. Cronin and K. Milgate. *A Vision of Future Health Care Delivery Systems: Organized Systems of Care.* (Washington, DC: Washington Business Group on Health, 1993).

10. Ibid.

11. M. Hammer and J. Champy. *Reengineering the Corporation: A Manifesto for Business Revolution* (New York: Harper Collins Publishers, 1993).

12. L. Curtin. *Nursing into the 21st Century* (Springhouse, PA: Springhouse Corporation, 1986), p. 270.

13. R. Farson. *Management of the Absurd: Paradoxes in Leadership* (New York: Simon & Schuster, 1996).

14. M. Wheatley. *Leadership and the New Science* (San Francisco: Berrett-Koehler Publishers, 1992).

15. Senge.

16. E. O. Bevis and J. Watson. *Toward a Caring Curriculum: A New Pedagogy for Nursing* (New York: National League for Nursing, 1989).

17. Curtin.

18. Porter-O'Grady and Wilson.

19. L. Loranger. Changing Health Care System Demands New Leaders, *Front & Center* 2, no. 3 (1998): 2–4.

20. D. D. Dubois. *Competency Based Performance Improvement: A Strategy for Organizational Improvement* (Amherst, MA: Human Resource Development Press, 1993).

21. C. K. Wilson. *Building New Nursing Organizations: Visions and Realities* (Gaithersburg, MD: Aspen Publishers, 1992).

22. Loranger, p. 4.

23. Wilson, p. 94.

24. J. T. Nilson. Life in the Middle: What It Takes to Succeed in Middle Management, *Healthcare Executive* (1998): 21–24.

25. J. M. Patz, D. L. Biordi, and K. Holm. Middle Manager Effectiveness, *JONA* 21, no. 1 (1991): 15–21.

26. Hammer and Champy.

27. E. C. Murphy and M. Snell. *The Genius of Sitting Bull: 13 Heroic Strategies for Today's Business Leaders* (Englewood Cliffs, NJ: Prentice-Hall, 1993).

28. R. Beckhard and W. Pritchard. *Changing the Essence* (San Francisco, Jossey-Bass Publishers, 1992), p. 65.

29. Ibid., p. 67.

30. D. Ulrich and D. Lake. *Organizational Capability: Competing from the Inside Out* (New York: John Wiley and Sons, 1990), p. 2.

Bibliography

Aroian, J., P. M. Meservey, and J. G. Crockett. Developing Nurse Leaders for Today and Tomorrow, *JONA* 26, no. 9 (1996): 18–26.

Bennis, W., and B. Nanus. *Leaders: The Strategies for Taking Charge* (New York: Harper and Row Publishers, 1985).

Kohles, M. K., W. G. Baker, and B. A. Donaho. *Transformational Leadership: Renewing Fundamental Values and Achieving New Relationships in Health Care* (Chicago: American Hospital Publishing, 1995).

McCrea, M. A. Personal Reflections on Early Learning in Shared Leadership, *Seminars for Nurse Managers* 6, no. 2 (1998): 83–88.

Morris, D., and J. Brandon. *Re-engineering Your Business* (New York: McGraw-Hill, 1993).

Sieloff, C. Nursing Leadership for a New Century, *Seminar for Nurse Managers* 4, no. 4 (1996): 226–33.

Stoner, James A, and R. E. Freeman. *Management*, 5th ed. (Englewood Cliffs, NJ: Prentice-Hall, 1992).

8

Nurses in the Marketplace: A Moral Option?

Laurence J. O'Connell, PhD, STD

I n the twentieth century, we experienced what Paul Starr called the social transformation of American medicine.[1] At the dawn of the twenty-first century, we are entering a period that promises another defining transformation of American medicine and, indeed, our entire health care system. In fact, the market transformation of health care is well under way. As we move into the next century, it is market competition rather than notions of human decency that will determine the direction of the U.S. health care system. Market forces will predominate in health care organization and delivery, while health care policy remains captive to a fundamentally manipulative political process. This is the (perhaps) sad but true state of affairs.

The provision of health care is contextual; that is, healers and those seeking healing derive their self-understanding and basic expectations respectively from a cultural context. Fundamental shifts in the environment inevitably alter self-perceptions and public expectations. As the competitive market has gained dominance as the preferred vehicle for reforming health care, for example, the popular view of medical practitioners has evolved. "From the mid-nineteenth century through the first half of the twentieth century, the cultural figure of the doctor evolved from a businessman to a professional. In the late twentieth century, the doctor has been reconceived as an entrepreneur who is now in the business of insuring patients as well as caring for them."[2] It should come as no surprise, then, that many doctors now sign off as MD, MBA.

This chapter looks at the role the nursing profession can play in ensuring ethical integrity in an increasingly market-driven health care system. To begin, the chapter describes the core features of the market concept and how they apply to the current health care environment.

THE HEALTH CARE MARKETPLACE

A comprehensive discussion of underlying economic theory or a spirited refutation of the market as an instrument of health reform would be out of place here. As interesting as these topics may be, they would distract from the central concern of this chapter: the vitality and integrity of the nursing profession in an entrepreneurial environment. However, some attention to the core features of the market concept is necessary as background.

Market is one of those weasel words that are capable of many twistings and turnings. Yet, the market concept does exhibit some fairly distinctive features that are shaping today's health care delivery system. Mark Peterson, in a special and very informative issue of the *Journal of Health Politics, Policy, and Law*, capsulizes these formative influences as follows:

- Private institutions regulate the flow of funds between payers and providers of care, although payers may be either private or public.
- Those private institutions promote payment mechanisms that use incentives to promote cost-effectiveness.
- Contracting is a dominant mode of establishing formal relationships between purchasers of coverage and insurers, between insurers and providers, among providers, and so on.
- For-profit firms are acceptable participants in health care.
- Despite federal and state regulations affecting individual and institutional behavior in the market, decisions about insurance products and the delivery of medical services are predominantly made by private actors.[3]

So what is the bottom line here? The prominence of three terms in the features outlined by Professor Peterson point the way. The terms *private*, *profit*, and *contract* represent the bright lines of market-driven reform. Private interests negotiate contractual agreements designed around incentives to control price and utilization while maximizing profitability.

This approach may well yield some economic advantages, at least in the short run. But some see in this the inevitable corporatization of health care, which will lead "to the commodification of medical services, with the conversion of patients into consumers and healers into entrepreneurs."[4] Others argue that this drive to commodify health and healing "diverts attention from the uninsured, the underinsured, and distributive equity to a concentrated focus on efficiency as defined by market forces. . . ."[5] They contend we are on our way to a moral train wreck.

In *The Wealth of Nations*, Adam Smith referred to "a propensity of human nature to exchange, . . . the propensity to truck, barter, and exchange one thing for another."[6] And, in the same context, Smith elaborated upon the uniquely human practice of making contracts for the purposes of fulfilling needs and wants. "Nobody ever saw one animal by its gestures and natural cries signify to another, this is mine, that yours; I am willing to give this for that."[7] Human behavior, however, exhibits a "trucking disposition," which seems to prefer meeting even basic needs through treaty, barter, and purchase. "It is not from the benevolence of the butcher, the brewer, or the baker that we expect our dinner, but from their regard to their own interest."[8] Here Smith lays bare the dynamic of the marketplace: "We address ourselves, not to their humanity but their self-love, and never talk to them of our own necessities but of their advantages."[9] The marketplace, with its emphasis on self-interest, is a morally ambiguous arena. The incentives to exploit, coerce, and engage in moral compromise are tightly woven into its fabric.

Again, our purpose in this context is not to offer an in-depth critique of the current state of health care organization and delivery. Having briefly described some salient features of the environment, we can move on to consider the place of the nursing profession in a market-oriented system. How can nurses engage in marketplace activities while retaining their traditional commitments to selfless caring for individuals and communities? The tensions are apparent, but they are not insurmountable.

NURSES AND THE MARKETPLACE

The nursing profession, of course, is not immune to the impact of market forces. It would be naive for the nursing professional to deny the realities of the marketplace or to pretend that in the current environment the profession can be free of commercial influence. Nurses, like physicians and other health care providers, must redefine their self-understanding in ways that will address market demands, while also ensuring the integrity of their professional calling.

The moral dangers associated with the need to derive personal gain from nursing activities have long been recognized. Since the early twentieth century, the traditional ideal that nursing should be untainted by financial considerations has evoked a degree of uneasiness. Tensions were already quite evident in the "early discussions of ethics in nursing between promoting patient welfare as a primary emphasis and promoting the welfare of nurses through adequate reimbursement. . . ."[10] Some form of economic exchange was part of the moral equation, albeit less prominent and powerful than it is today, narrowly confined to the issue of a just wage. Currently, however, nurses have been swept into a much broader economic arena that links them inextricably with the marketplace. Today's environment harshly exposes an uneasy truth: nursing is indeed a vocation, but it is also an enterprise wherein professional identity, moral agency, and social responsibility simply cannot avoid commercial influence and marketplace dynamics. In short, the nursing profession does not exist in a moral vacuum. How, then, does nursing make its way in the marketplace?

In seeking a responsible and morally credible response, two fundamental questions must be addressed:

1.   Are the workings of a competitive, private enterprise economy morally defective and ethically unacceptable in the realm of health care?
2.   Should it be determined that a marketplace orientation is not absolutely out of place, how can the nursing profession retain a sense of vocation and commitment to traditional values while negotiating its way through the grand bazaar of managed care?

Questioning the Moral Tenor of the Marketplace

In answer to the first question above, it can be asserted that the marketplace is not inherently evil. What people do within the context of a market-oriented economy and social service system may indeed be morally wrong. But ultimately the moral tenor of marketplace activities is dependent upon the moral agency of individuals, organizations, and societies at large. While an undiscriminating and uncritical endorsement of market-oriented approaches to the distribution of goods and services would be naive, an outright condemnation of competitive, cost-conscious enterprise would be equally simplistic. Of course, unrestricted free competition that allows the survival of only those who are strongest is morally repugnant. But the market model need not give way to the greed of unbridled competition. In principle, it should be possible to harmonize the demands of the marketplace with the moral requirements of justice and the common good.

Such harmonization, though, can be difficult and elusive in practice—especially in an area like health care. Whether this kind of harmonization is possible at all is the subject of some debate. "Many, if not most, health economists believe that the competitive model is an appropriate means for studying (and perhaps reforming) health care systems."[11] Yet, there are persuasive detractors among the economists who reject the supposed superiority of market competition in the health care area "because the competitive model is based upon certain assumptions that do not appear to be met."[12]

Ethicists also have entered the fray. Some argue that market-driven reform is morally admissible, while others reject the new paradigm as bad medicine. In conclusion, then, it is difficult to dismiss current market-driven forces in health care as absolutely wrong-headed. Whether the economic theory can bear the weight of implementation in the practical order remains to be seen. And, more important, whether the emerging system can meet the moral requirements of justice and the common good is still open to serious question.

However, the fact is that although the market-based approach to health care organization, delivery, and financing may be highly suspect in both economic and ethical terms, there is little likelihood that it will disappear any time soon. In a populace resistant to government intervention and deeply marked by an individualistic spirit in economic affairs, market mechanisms will continue to find favor until they are either proven hopelessly ineffective or occasion serious social unrest and political upheaval. These conditions are unlikely to develop until some time in the new century. As a result, nurses, like other health care professionals, will be squarely situated in the marketplace for some time to come.

Moreover, the marketplace may be morally messy, but for now it is the principal venue for effective action. Until social priorities and public policy shift, market forces will continue to shape health care organization, finance, and delivery. Inactive longing and ineffectual desire for a morally perfect world will do little to advance the legitimate interests of nursing at this point in history. And fleeing the marketplace is not an option!

Questioning the Nursing Role

Given the circumstances discussed above in response to the first question, what is the answer to the second question with regard to today's nurses retaining a sense of vocation and personal integrity while seeking an appropriate and morally influential role in the marketplace? As a point of departure, it is important to remember that all persons, institutions, and societies are capable of doing both good and evil. Indeed, the moral life comprises a struggle to do the least harm while doing the most good. Unfortunately, though, the good we do is often at a cost. In ethical reflection we seek practical wisdom and guidance in an effort to maximize good while limiting the potentially—and often unavoidable—bad side effects of our actions. To be ethical in the marketplace, then, is not to be morally blameless. It is rather to do our very best to achieve good while avoiding as much evil as possible in a morally murky environment.

Of course, there must be personal, institutional, and social limits on the degree and extent of bad side effects. Although it may be legal, for example, physicians cannot be forced on the personal level to euthanize patients, Catholic hospitals cannot be compelled to terminate pregnancies, and the U.S. government will not allow certain forms of human experimentation. Clearly, then, individuals, institutions, and society at large sketch moral boundaries that define their place in today's health care marketplace. Each health care provider and institution operates, either implicitly or explicitly, according to a moral vision of marketplace participation. To the degree that each participant in the morally ambiguous marketplace attends to its ethical character, the chances for good outcomes will be immeasurably improved. Indeed, a proactive choice by professionals to enter the marketplace may demand moral compromise, but it also presents an opportunity to inject a degree of ethical sensitivity that can curb the greed of unrestrained competition.

Thus, the fact that nurses work in the marketplace does not necessarily mean they must betray their personal or professional values. Indeed, at times they must make compromises in favor of what may be the lesser good; but that is an inescapable by-product of a market-driven environment. As noted earlier, nurses do not exist in a moral vacuum. They are subject to the social conditions, moral complexities, and ethical shortcomings of the world they inhabit. Consequently, nurses cannot escape the morally ambiguous dynamics of the health care marketplace. Heart, soul, and body, they are enmeshed in the dealings of this entrepreneurial day and age.

Drawing upon her knowledge of nursing practice, Mae Moss provides a common yet telling example:

> In the classic case of an aging patient who requires long-term inpatient care, the patient's economic status [market value] dictates whether that care is a function of ethical decision making. If the family has resources [private capital] for continued care, no ethical decision exists [at least not with reference to payment for services]. However, if the family is uninsured or has limited resources, the nurse may be faced with a possible situation in which treatment allocation [funds available for a specific case] borders on health care rationing [funds available for an entire population]. In this case, the family's income level [buying power], the institution's policies [regarding inability to pay], and the national economics of managed care [cost containment] all influence the outcome.[13] (Bracketed material added)

This case suggests the broad range of moral challenges arising within market-driven health care where, as previously noted, private interests negotiate contractual agreements designed around incentives to control price and utilization while maximizing financial returns. Parenthetically, it should be noted that this dynamic applies to both for-profit and not-for-profit health care systems in the United States. Although their respective uses of financial returns are different, they both participate in the marketplace to generate those returns. In short, the moral vagaries of the marketplace play out in both for-profit and not-for-profit enterprises.

In the case described above, the nurse confronts ethical issues on several levels simultaneously. Is she being asked to violate her moral duty towards the well-being of her vulnerable patient? Is she morally responsible for protecting the financial viability of the institution? Does she have an ethical duty as a citizen to promote justice in the allocation of health care resources? Although this case points to the complexity of doing good and avoiding evil in a market-driven health care system, it also contains hints about a constructive, ethically sensitive response to the inevitable moral quandaries, discussed next.

NURSES AS ADVOCATES FOR THE COMMON GOOD

Given their pivotal role, nurses are uniquely positioned to serve as advocates for the common good within a market-oriented health care delivery system. Nurse practitioners, nurse managers, and nurse policy analysts intersect with just about every dimension of the health care system. Their level of engagement moves out from the bedside through corporate and governance functions to public health initiatives and public policy work. The pervasive presence of the nursing profession places it in close proximity to the complex professional, organizational, and social forces that currently shape health care financing and delivery. Through day-to-day contact with these forces, the nursing profession can play a significant role in drawing attention to the moral and ethical dimensions of an environment that has been characterized as "balkanized, profit-crazed, unguided, and unintelligible."[14]

Nurses can help ensure the ethical integrity of the health care system on at least three levels of engagement:

- *On the personal level*, nurses can influence the morality of the marketplace through personal vigilance and exercise of their duty to protect and advocate for their patients.
- *On the institutional level*, nurses can exercise moral accountability for the expenditure of resources essential to the viability of their institution.
- *On the social level*, as knowledgeable citizens, nurses can actively think about the moral implications of resource deployment in the current health care system and serve as social advocates.

Personal, institutional, and social moral concerns collide in a powerful way. The incentives of the marketplace subtly—or maybe not so subtly—shape the moral contours of the nurse's experience, her patient's care, and society's response to those in need. Nurses, then, can influence the morality of the marketplace through personal vigilance, institutional management, and social advocacy. But there is more.

As nurses begin to address unmet market demand for nursing services, they will be drawn into the gray zone of entrepreneurial activity. They will not be passive observers as they give care, manage services, or advocate for change; rather, they will be active brokers in a market-driven system. They will begin to structure independent business initiatives and enter into complex partnerships. This active posture will definitely require moral trade-offs. And herein lies the challenge.

CONCLUSION

As the world of health care adapts to the demands of the marketplace, so too must nursing find innovative ways and means to survive and compete with integrity. As discussed in this chapter, a market-oriented approach is not inherently evil. The moral quality of marketplace activities is dependent upon the moral agency of individuals, organizations, and societies at large. The current situation provides an opportunity for the nursing profession to play a larger social role. Through ethically attuned enterprise in service provision, nurse practitioners, managers, and entrepreneurs can lead the way in harmonizing the demands of the marketplace with the moral requirements of justice and the common good. Although the crucible of market-oriented reform will radically reshape large segments of the nursing profession, it need not destroy its integrity. The moral life is just that—life! Inanimate systems can more or less support the deepest aspirations of the human spirit, but only people can make those systems more or less good. The traditional moral commitments of the nursing profession can and will survive the age of market-driven health care; but the overall success in the near term will depend on the practical ingenuity and moral imagination of nurses themselves. Nurses in the marketplace? Undoubtedly a moral option and definitely a welcome addition!

References

1. Paul Starr, *The Social Transformation of American Medicine* (New York: Basic Books, 1982).

2. Deborah A. Stone. The Doctor as Businessman: The Changing Politics of a Cultural Icon, *Journal of Health Politics, Policy, and Law* 22, no. 2 (1997): 534.

3. Mark A. Peterson. Introduction: Health Care into the Next Century, *Journal of Health Politics, Policy, and Law* 22, no. 2 (1997): 303–4.

4. Ibid., 299.

5. Ibid., 300.

6. Adam Smith. *An Inquiry into the Nature and Causes of the Wealth of Nations*, Edwin Cannan, ed. (Chicago, IL: University of Chicago Press, 1976), p. 17.

7. Ibid., p. 18.

8. Ibid.

9. Ibid.

10. Mila Ann Aroskar. Ethics in Nursing and Health Care Reform: Back to the Future? *Hastings Center Report* 24, no. 3 (1994): 11.

11. Thomas Rice. Can Markets Give Us the Health Care System We Want?" *Journal of Health Politics, Policy, and Law* 22, no. 2 (1997): 387.

12. Ibid., p. 396.

13. Mae Taylor Moss. Principles, Values, and Ethics Set the Stage for Managed Care Nursing, *Nursing Economic$* 13, no. 5 (1995): 279.

14. Robert Reno. Health Care Reform Failed, but a Revolution Happened Anyway, *Cedar Rapids Gazette* (June 25, 1997): 4A.

Index